Skin Cancer:
A Practical Guide
to Management

Graham B Colver DM FRCP FRCPE

Consultant Dermatologist
Royal Hospital
Calow
Chesterfield
UK

With contributions from

Bill Bowers
Robert Burd
Catriona Irvine
Peter Kersey
Clifford Lawrence
Jerry Marsden
Graeme Stables
Nicholas Telfer

Martin Dunitz

© 2002 Martin Dunitz Ltd,
a member of the Taylor & Francis group

First published in the United Kingdom in 2002
by Martin Dunitz Ltd, The Livery House, 7–9 Pratt Street,
London NW1 0AE

Tel.: +44 (0) 20 74822202
Fax.: +44 (0) 20 72670159
E-mail: info@dunitz.co.uk
Website: http://www.dunitz.co.uk

A CIP record for this book is available from the British Library.

ISBN 1 84184 173 0

Distributed in the USA by
Fulfilment Center
Taylor & Francis
7625 Empire Drive
Florence, KY 41042, USA
Toll Free Tel.: +1 800 634 7064
E-mail: cserve@routledge_ny.com

Distributed in Canada by
Taylor & Francis
74 Rolark Drive
Scarborough, Ontario M1R 4G2, Canada
Toll Free Tel.: +1 877 226 2237
E-mail: tal_fran@istar.ca

Distributed in the rest of the world by
Thomson Publishing Services
Cheriton House
North Way
Andover, Hampshire SP10 5BE, UK
Tel.: +44 (0)1264 332424
E-mail: salesorder.tandf@thomsonpublishingservices.co.uk

Composition by Scribe Design, Gillingham, Kent, UK
Printed and bound in Singapore by Kyodo Printing Co (S'pore) Pte Ltd

Contents

Contributors

Bill Bowers FRCP
Consultant Dermatologist
Department of Dermatology
Royal Cornwall Hospitals Trust
Truro
Cornwall
UK

Robert Burd
Consultant Dermatologist
Leicester Royal Infirmary
Leicester
UK

Catriona Irvine
William Harvey Hospital
Ashford
Kent
UK

Peter Kersey
Consultant Dermatologist
Department of Dermatology
Derriford Hospital
Plymouth
UK

Clifford Lawrence MD FRCP
Consultant Dermatologist
Skin Department
Royal Victoria Infirmary
Newcastle-upon-Tyne
UK

Jerry Marsden
Department of Dermatology
University Hospital NHS Trust
Selly Oak Hospital
Birmingham
UK

Graeme Stables MBChB MD MRCP
Consultant Dermatologist
Department of Dermatology
The United Leeds Teaching Hospitals
UK

Nicholas Telfer FRCP
Consultant Dermatologist
Dermatology Centre
Hope Hospital
Salford
UK

Foreword

Skin cancer is now fully recognized as a serious public health problem. A significant number of people die from melanoma each year and even more suffer through the disfiguring effects of the much more prevalent non-melanoma skin cancers. This is glaringly brought to our attention by the media each time a ranking politician or famous entertainer is afflicted. As almost all of these skin tumours are related to over-exposure to the ultraviolet rays in sunshine, they appear most often on the sun-exposed face, neck or upper extremities. Almost all the rest appear on the intermittently exposed skin of the back, chest and lower extremities. Beside the significant mortality, the time lost from work, the expense to the health system and the anguish caused by being a cancer victim is staggering.

It is imperative that the public be educated about early recognition and primary preventative strategies. And it is equally important that primary care physicians are aware of the scope of the problem, that they develop diagnostic skills and are trained either be able to perform appropriate biopsy for histological examination or to refer to a dermatologist for diagnosis and/or management. Finally, dermatologists must be fully trained in the full range of issues attendant to skin cancers; their recognition, the available diagnostic procedures, the management strategies and the full scope of treatment procedures. Dermatologists must have, in addition to these skills, an ability to educate the press, the public and the primary care physician. They must also act as part of a multi-disciplinary team in the care of complicated tumours. This book fulfils all these missions in a well organized, succinct, easy to read and beautifully illustrated manner. There are inevitably considerable differences in the approach to managing skin cancers in different countries. They relate to the organization of the health services, patient preferences in different societies and the prevalence of difficult tumours in fair skinned individuals living in subtropical climates.

There are differences, between countries, in the nature of the specialty that treats the majority of skin cancers. In the USA and much of Europe surgical dermatologists have had this role for a long time whereas in the UK dermatologists have been increasing their surgical repertoire over the last twenty years. Worldwide there has been a greater emphasis on surgical procedures during residency training and there are many opportunities for advanced Surgical Fellowship training. Hence, there is a strong surgical infrastructure across the country and in the USA micrographic surgery is available in almost every community. However in any country the importance for patients is whether an expert who has knowledge of all the available modalities, who uses them appropriately and who has high cure rates with good cosmetic results, treats them.

The message in this book is universal and commensurate with good medicine anywhere in the world. While professing to cover areas crucial to good patient management, it is this and much more.

Stuart J. Salasche, MD
Clinical Professor, University of Arizona
Health Sciences Center
Research Scientist, Cancer Center, University
of Arizona Health Sciences Center, USA

Introduction

Skin cancer is visible and common. There is now so much publicity about the hazards of excess sun exposure and the tell tale signs of skin cancer that few people can have escaped the impact of the campaigns. These warnings bring more people to health care professionals but at the same time cause anxiety and many people have a distorted view of the risks, the relevance of moles and what it means if skin cancer is diagnosed. Part of the misunderstanding lies in the biological diversity of skin cancer. Not only are there three chief types - basal cell, squamous cell and melanoma - but the behaviour and aggressiveness of each type can vary widely between individuals. The recognition and appropriate management of this spectrum of malignant disease is the subject of this book. There are sections on education, prevention, aetiology, clinical and laboratory diagnosis. Priority is given to the principles of treatment but technical aspects are also covered with an emphasis on appropriateness for the different modalities. This is not a surgical manual but rather a dissertation on areas which are crucial to good patient management.

All of the authors are members of the British Society for Dermatological Surgery, which is affiliated to the British Association of Dermatologists. They have given freely of their time and each has contributed to more than one chapter. The book represents a distillation of the views of these authors who are all involved in busy clinical practice dealing with hundreds of cases of skin cancer each year. Dr Stuart Salasche, a prominent dermatological surgeon in America, has written a foreword highlighting the importance of skin cancer and the need for its appropriate management. In both countries dermatologists are the usual specialist point of referral for suspected and actual skin malignancy - for many of them dealing with skin tumours forms the majority of their work.

At the time this book was conceived the Therapy Guidelines Committee of the British Association of Dermatologists (BAD) had commissioned members to produce guidelines on the management of Bowen's disease, basal cell and squamous cell carcinoma and malignant melanoma. Several of the authors have contributed to this book. The manuscripts were sent to all dermatologists in the United Kingdom (and many other experts in the case of the melanoma document). We are grateful to the BAD for allowing us to include the guidelines as appendices to this book . The style of the guidelines is evidence based but complements the less proscriptive style of this book.

The book is aimed at all doctors who deal with skin cancer whether in primary, secondary or tertiary care. We hope that it will also give insight to nurses and other health care professionals working in dermatology and skin cancer departments.

Graham Colver
Editor

Acknowledgements

The nine contributors to this book are all members of the British Society for Dermatological Surgery (BSDS). The society aims to improve the knowledge and skills of all those involved in skin surgery. It runs annual practical workshops, a newsletter and academic days at the annual meeting. It also offers travelling fellowships to its members who wish to improve the breadth of their training. None of the authors received a fee for their contribution to this book and all of the royalties which accrue from its publication are going to the BSDS to further promote good practice in surgical dermatology

The Guidelines which are included as appendices were commissioned by the Therapy Guidelines Committee of the British Association of Dermatologists (BAD). These guidelines have been published in the British Journal of Dermatology and we are grateful to the BAD for permission to reproduce them here.

The members of the Therapy Guidelines Committee overseeing the publications on Bowen's disease, basal cell carcinoma and squamous cell carcinoma were CEM Griffiths, CB Bunker, SM Burge, NH Cox, CA Holden, MR Judge, DK Mehta, HC Williams; and for the melanoma guidelines NH Cox, AV Anstey, CB Bunker, MJD Goodfield, AS Highet, D Mehta, RH Meyrick Thomas and JK Schofield. The multiprofessional skin cancer committee representing the BAD, British Association of Plastic Surgeons and Faculty of Clinical Oncology of the Royal College of Radiologists were NH Cox, AY Finlay, BR Allen D Murray, RW Griffiths, A Batchelor, D Morgan, DK Schofield, CB Bunker, NR Telfer, GB Colver, PW Bowers and the authors.

The authors of the guidelines for Bowen's disease were NH Cox, DJ Eady, CA Morton. For basal cell carcinoma the authors were NR Telfer, GB Colver, PW Bowers. For squamous cell carcinoma the authors were R Motley, P Kersey, C Lawrence. For melanoma the authors were DLL Roberts, AV Anstey, RJ Barlo, NH Cox, JA Newton Bishop, PG Corrie, J Evans, ME Gore, PN Hall, N Kirkham.

1 About skin cancer

Skin cancer is the most common human malignancy and its incidence is rising more quickly than any other tumour. It is so well known that most people have some knowledge of the disease and its importance. It was one of the earliest cancers to be recognized and some of the first work which helped our understanding of cancer pathogenesis was with cutaneous squamous carcinoma. The external location of this cancer makes it amenable to detailed observation and biopsy and finally skin cancer has led to a huge literature studying the benefits of public education in the prevention of malignancy.

In most countries the incidence of skin cancer has shown a sharp increase over the last 15 years and this trend is expected to continue for several more years despite public awareness, education and prevention strategies. Malignant melanoma (MM) has a higher mortality than the nonmelanoma skin cancers (NMSCs) – basal cell and squamous cell. But MM is less common affecting approximately 15/100 000 in the UK each year compared to 80/100 000 for NMSCs. This book concentrates on these three tumours, but it is important to remember that any of the 20 or more cell types in the skin can produce malignant proliferation. These are dealt with in Chapter 6 together with mention of tumours which metastasize to the skin and some which invade the skin from adjacent tissues.

Size of the problem

Skin cancer and its ramifications are beginning to overwhelm current specialist services. The increasing incidence of the tumours is only one of the reasons. The population is ageing and malignant diseases of many types are seen with increasing frequency. More individuals are immunocompromised as a result of organ transplantation, medication and AIDS and they are at greatly increased risk of skin cancer which may also be particularly aggressive. Added to these factors the general public has increasingly high expectations of the National Health Service and is better informed, having ready access to global information systems through the Internet and other technology.

General practitioners, as the clinicians in primary care groups, are the first to see patients who are concerned about suspected skin cancer. However many nonspecialists have difficulty with dermatological diagnoses. This is in part because early skin cancer can be hard to differentiate from benign lesions but also because there is now less teaching of dermatology at medical school than at any time in the past. It takes trainees in dermatology many months of supervised work to become confident in diagnosis and management of suspected skin cancer so it is not surprising that many general practitioners, who may have had no such supervised training, tend to refer so much to the hospital.

Historical background

The earliest descriptions of skin cancer were of slow inexorable growths destroying all in their path. The Latin term – *noli me tangere* (touch me not) was given because they were thought to be incurable and therefore not to be treated. Even in the early nineteenth century skin ulcers of all aetiologies were often confused and no attempt was made to distinguish them. In 1775 Percival Pott made a detailed description of what we now call squamous carcinoma, but he did not use the term cancer. Possibly the first record of definite skin cancer was from Jacob in 1827, who recorded in the Dublin hospital journal 'an ulcer of peculiar character which attacks the eyelids and other parts of the face'. The term *ulcus rodens* was used in 1851, and two years later Sir James Paget referred to rodent ulcer. However some authors confused the entity with lupus vulgaris, syphilitic gumma and squamous carcinoma. By the 1860s most doctors realized that rodent ulcer and *noli me tangere* were the same and that they represented a type of skin cancer. The development of microscopes enabled the subject to advance and in 1865, Thiersch wrote that the tumour developed from the direct proliferation of the epithelioid elements. Twenty years later the concept of superficial (rodent ulcer) and deep (squamous cell) skin cancer appeared and in 1903, Krompecher wrote his monograph *Der Basalzellkrebs* (basal cell carcinoma).

Early descriptions of skin cancers

These cases describe the natural history of the three most common skin tumours. It is excep-tional to see anything like this today. There are still individuals who neglect their tumours, sometimes because they have a fear of doctors and hospital, or because they have a mental illness or occasionally because religious beliefs prevent them from accepting modern medical treatment. Apart from these situations, most people are seen early in the development of the tumour growth and remedial action is taken. These extracts also remind us of the extra-ordinary descriptive powers of many early physicians.

Squamous cell carcinoma (the chimney sweepers' cancer) – Percival Pott (1775)

It is a disease which always makes its first attack on, and its first appearance in the inferior part of the scrotum; where it produces a superficial painful, ragged, ill-looking sore, with hard and rising edges. The trade calls it the soot-wart. I never saw it under the age of puberty, which is, I suppose, one reason, why it is generally taken, both by patient and surgeon, for venereal, and being treated with mercurials, is thereby soon, and much exasperated: in no great length of time it pervades the skin, dartos, and membranes of the scrotum, and seizes the testicles, which it enlarges, hardens and renders truly and thoroughly distempered; from whence it makes its way up the spermatic process into the abdomen, most frequently indurating, and spoiling the inguinal glands: when arrived within the abdomen, it affects some of the viscera, and then very soon becomes painfully destructive … If there be any chance of putting a stop to, or preventing this mischief, it must be by the immediate removal of the part affected. I mean the part of the scrotum where the sore is, for if it be suffered to remain until the virus has seized the testicle, it is generally too late even for castration. I have many times made the experiment; but though the sores, after such operation, have, in some instances, healed kindly, and the patients have gone from the hospital seemingly well, yet, in the space of a few months, it has generally happened, that they have returned either with the same disease in the other testicle, or in the glands from the groin, or with such wan complexions, such pale, leaden, countenances, such a total loss of strength, and such frequent and acute internal pains, as have sufficiently proved a diseased state of some of the viscera, and which have soon been followed by a painful death.

Malignant melanoma – William Norris (1820)

Mr ... aged 59, apparently in good health applied to me in consequence of the inconvenience he felt from a tumour, situated nearly mid-way between the umbilicus and pubes. He told me there had always been a mole exactly in the same spot, and that nine months ago, the skin around this congenital mark assumed a brownish hue and that from the part thus discoloured the tumour began to arise. On examination, I found the swelling was nearly of half the size of a hens egg, of a deep brown colour, of a firm and fleshy feel, ulcerated on its surface, which discharged a highly fetid ichorous fluid. The apex of the tumour was broader than its base. Some few months after the appearance of this tumour, distinct nodules sprung up around it, some with slender necks, others with broader bases. This singular production was at length removed by the knife, and the wound went on favourably, and healed. In less than six weeks the tumour again began to grow from the cicatrised

surface, and felt hard and semi-cartilaginous, and very soon minute tubercles, of a livid colour, surrounded the tumour; some of them separated from, and others growing into, each other. Of the latter sort there were at least forty in number, forming a mass of disease extending nearly from the spine of one os ileum to the other, and bearing a resemblance to a large bunch of dark-coloured grapes, some of them flattened on the surface, and of various sizes. The prominent scirrhous-looking tumour occupied the centre; the tubercles already formed progressively increased, while fresh ones arose in their vicinity. The glands in the groin were swollen, and slightly tender to the touch.

This disorganisation of parts was effected in two months, and continued to increase after that period. Bluish spots arose in the vicinity of a mole upon the sternum; others appeared in succession on the sides of the body, and on the back; and very soon the forehead and scalp were disfigured with the same morbid appearances. The animal frame became perceptibly impaired, and the patient very soon unable to leave his bed-room. Symptoms of general dropsy had for some weeks shown themselves, and these were soon followed by an increase of restlessness, cough, and difficulty of breathing, until death closed his miserable existence.

Appearance after Death

'When the abdomen, chest and cranium were thrown open, it was a most extrodinary phenomenon; thousands of circular shapes and various sizes, were to be seen closely dotting the shining mucous, serous and fibrous membranes of most of the vital organs; I should think the most dazzling sight ever beheld by a morbid anatomist. I shall never forget the pleasing thrill that came over me when I first beheld them. It would have puzzled the most powerful descriptive talent *to have done full justice to such a novel and striking disease, displayed so beautifully in endless profusion everywhere.*

Rodent ulcer – Arthur Jacob (1827)

I allude to a destructive ulceration of peculiar character, which I have observed to attack and destroy the eyelids, and extend to the eyeball, orbit and face. The characteristic features of this disease are, the extraordinary slowness of its progress, the peculiar condition of the edges and surface of the ulcer, the comparatively inconsiderable suffering produced by it, its incurable nature unless by extirpation, and its not contaminating the neighbouring lymphatic glands. The slowness with which this disease proceeds is very remarkable. The edges are elevated, smooth and glossy, with a serpentine outline; and are occasionally formed into a range of small tubercles or elevations: the skin in the vicinity is not thickened or discoloured. The part within the edges is in some places a perfectly smooth, vascular, secreting surface, having veins of considerable size ramifying over it; which veins occasionally give way, causing slight haemorrhage; in other places the surface appears covered by florid healthy looking granulations, firm in texture and remaining unchanged in size and form for a great length of time. The surface sometimes even heals over in patches, which are hard, smooth and marked with the venous ramifications to which I have alluded.

There is no inconsiderable bleeding from the surface, and when it does occur, it arises from the superficial veins giving way, and not from sloughing or ulceration opening vessels; sometimes the surface assumes a dark gangrenous appearance, which I have found to arise from the effusion of blood beneath. I have not observed that the lymphatic glands were in the slightest degree contaminated, the disease being altogether extended by ulceration from the point from whence it commences.

It remains to be determined whether this disease can be removed by any other means than the knife or powerful escharotics; and from the experience I have had in those cases, I am inclined to conclude that it bids defiance to all remedies short of extirpation. I have observed that one of those cases which is completely neglected, and left without any other dressing other than a piece of rag, is slower in its progress than another which has had all the resources of surgery exhausted upon it.

Public health

The incidence of the three main types of skin cancer is increasing. It is possible that some of this increase may be a pseudo-epidemic due to increased reporting but on the other hand official cancer registration statistics probably underestimate the incidence. A recent survey in Trent region suggested that 25% of melanoma are not registered and an earlier survey in Bristol that between 14 and 28% of NMSC was unregistered in 1974. Yet it is still the commonest form of cancer in the UK. An important reason for consistently underestimating the incidence of skin cancer is that registers do not record patients with second primaries – some patients have multiple tumours. Recently some centres have ceased to record NMSC altogether with the result that any future data will have to come from hospital databases.

Overall the incidence of NMSC appears to have approximately doubled between 1980 and 1990. In the UK it is approximately 80/100 000. This is due to increased occupational and recreational exposure to ultraviolet radiation, increased longevity and the depleted ozone layer. The realization that this trend represented a significant health problem was officially recognized by the inclusion of skin cancer in the Health of the Nation document in 1992 and the Europe Against Cancer Campaign. The stated target in the Health of the Nation document was 'to halt the year on year increase in the incidence of skin cancer by 2005'. This is a commendable target even if the aetiological and epidemiological factors mean that it may not be achievable in such a short timespan. Since 1993, skin cancer public health messages have been co-ordinated by a National UK Skin Cancer Working Party representing dermatologists, cancer charities and the Health Education Council. It deals with four separate areas:

● cancer registration problems,
● helping the primary care team,
● helping hospital skin cancer services,
● public education.

Each year a Sun Know How campaign is launched targeted at specific groups to push home the messages about reducing exposure to ultraviolet radiation.

Educating the public about sun avoidance is fairly new in the UK but has been a major exercise in Australia for much longer. The Australians have led the world in the area of public education. Their incidence of skin cancer is approximately 10 times higher than in the UK and reflects the lifestyle of a fair skinned race living in low latitudes.

Economic impact

Melanoma accounted for 1142 deaths in England and Wales in 1992. Approximately 25% of people will eventually die of their disease. On the other hand very few people die from the more common NMSC which has a 5-year survival rate of nearly 97% and a ratio of incidence to mortality around 160:1. For the most part NMSC is a disease simply treated by day care surgery. A few patients may require radiotherapy and some with difficult tumours may require a general anaesthetic and a short hospital stay. Metastatic NMSC is uncommon but may require further admission for surgery.

The treatment of primary melanoma is surgical and in some cases lymph node dissection is also needed. Melanoma treatment may be very expensive if metastatic disease occurs. Surgery, investigations and chemotherapy or immunotherapy all contribute to a costly package of care.

Public campaigns, which encourage the public to seek advice about changing lesions, have a considerable economic impact. It is unlikely that a GP will acquire sufficient expertise to safely exclude melanoma on clinical grounds, so it falls to the hospital services to offer this service. Without this expertise, unnecessary surgery and much patient anxiety are inevitable.

Who deals with skin cancer?

Currently skin cancer is diagnosed and managed by primary care physicians, dermatologists and surgeons in several specialties. Historically dermatologists have always played a central role. This situation has applied in Europe and the USA for over a century. Founders of dermatology in the UK had as often been surgeons as physicians. Erasmus Wilson, Jonathan Paget and Jonathan Hutchinson are examples and

Erasmus Wilson in his own college – the Royal College of Surgeons – founded the first chair of dermatology.

Dermatologists are usually the first point of referral for skin cancer and suspected skin cancer for several reasons.

- They have played a key role in education of the public concerning the hazards of ultraviolet exposure and the need for assessment of changing lesions.
- They were involved in the early developments of clinics devoted to the assessment of pigmented or changing lesions – together with outpatient facilities geared towards immediate biopsy or excision of suitable lesions.
- They have extensive training in diagnosis, understanding the biological behaviour of skin cancer and premalignant diseases and in clinico-pathological correlation. There is evidence that for melanoma, dermatologists are more likely to enter the correct diagnosis on the pathology form than plastic surgeons[1] and to diagnose melanoma more accurately than nondermatologists.[2] General practitioners made a confident diagnosis of melanoma in only 17% of patients prior to surgery.[3] However, in other studies amongst dermatologists, the senior staff with more than 10 years' experience had a significantly greater diagnostic accuracy than junior members. Finally, in a plastic surgery unit doctors seeing a lot of melanoma had a high rate of correct diagnoses. Whoever is given the task of diagnosing pigmented lesions must have a wealth of clinical experience.
- They have training in a variety of surgical procedures including excisional surgery, curettage and cryosurgery. This range allows the most appropriate modality to

be used in individual cases.
- They are the chief exponents of the exacting technique of micrographic surgery.

Dermatologists are the main point of referral for suspected skin cancer. Diagnostic biopsy may be required or one of the many treatment modalities may be used without prior biopsy. At least 90% of skin cancers are treated by dermatologists especially those with a special interest in dermatological surgery. Not all geographical areas will have an experienced dermatological surgeon and in these localities other surgical specialists will deal with the bulk of the tumours. Large and deeply infiltrating tumours, those with nodal metastases or requiring complex reconstruction will more often be seen by specialists in plastic or oculoplastic surgery, ENT, maxillofacial surgery, radiotherapy and oncology. Often a multidisciplinary approach is needed.

Provision of skin cancer services

Recently attempts have been made to clarify the pathways for referral and management of skin cancer as part of the National Policy Framework for Commissioning Cancer Services. The general principles underlying the provision of these services (as for all cancers) across the UK have been formulated. They include

- access to uniformly high quality of care,
- education to promote early recognition,
- clear information about treatment options,
- patient centred approach,
- recognition of the psychosocial aspect of cancer care,

- effective cancer registration and monitoring treatment outcomes.

The new structure is based on a network of expertise in cancer care reaching from primary care through cancer units in district hospitals to cancer centres. Cancer units are being created in most district general hospitals with responsibility for guidelines of referral, multidisciplinary expertise and good communication with both primary care and the cancer centres. The volume of work must be great enough to maintain subspecialist expertise. The cancer centres will be one or more large hospitals, which can offer services such as radiotherapy, chemotherapy, complex reconstructive surgery, new techniques and possible multicentre trials of new treatments.

A set of standards has been widely distributed covering many aspects of care. Multidisciplinary team working will be mandatory and a record of all team decisions documented so that the data can be audited at a later stage. During the latter part of 2000 hospitals were assessed by accreditation teams to ensure that all the standards were being met.

References

1. Williams HC, Smith D, du Vivier A (1991) Melanoma. Differences observed by general surgeons and dermatologists, *Int J Dermatol* **30**:257–61.
2. Kopf AW, Minzis M, Bart RS (1975) Diagnostic accuracy in malignant melanoma, *Arch Dermatol* **111**:1291–2.
3. Khorshid SM, Pinney E, Bishop JA (1998) Melanoma excision by general practitioners in north-east Thames region, England, *Br J Dermatol* **138**:412–7.

2 Precancer

What is precancer?

The term precancer or premalignancy implies a condition of the skin or mucous membrane which, if left untreated, may eventually become malignant. There is no exact definition which helps to distinguish between very rare occurrences, such as malignant change in a seborrhoeic keratosis, and more frequent events such as transformation of Bowen's disease (BD) into a squamous carcinoma. There is mention in this chapter of the concept that solar keratosis, BD and lentigo maligna (LM) are in fact already malignant but in situ. These are the three conditions dealt with here. It is important to note that other diseases have an accepted risk of malignant change. On mucosal surfaces the main examples are leukoplakia, lichen sclerosus and erosive lichen planus. On the skin they include areas damaged by ionizing or infrared radiation, keratoses induced by tar or inorganic arsenic compounds and long-standing areas of chronic inflammation such as sinuses, scars, tuberculosis and ulcers.

Actinic keratosis

Introduction

Actinic keratosis (AK) is a common sun-induced premalignant neoplasm of the epidermis that occurs primarily on exposed skin. The first mention of AK appeared in 1894 when Unna described them in his treatise *Carcinom der Seemannshaut* ('sea-man's skin'). Actinic keratosis has been known by many names (actinic keratosis, solar keratosis, senile keratosis and senile hyperkeratosis). Actinic (from Greek *aktis* meaning ray) keratosis or solar keratosis are preferred names as they convey information about both aetiology and appearance. Senile keratosis or senile hyperkeratosis should be avoided, as there may be confusion with seborrhoeic keratosis also known as senile wart. Also the inclusion of the word senile obscures the fact that actinic keratosis is related more to sun exposure than age.

There are two viewpoints on the malignant status of AK. One places it as a pathological change at the mildly dysplastic end of a clinical and histological continuum that progresses to invasive squamous cell carcinoma (SCC). However there is a strong and valid argument that AK is squamous carcinoma in the same way that BD is SCC and melanoma in situ is melanoma. Most clinicians are happy with this as a concept but it does not make patient management easy. It is easier to manage patients on the basis that they have a premalignant condition and to explain that only when the basement membrane has been breached has the lesion become malignant. Some of the sections in this chapter, such as those on differential diagnosis and risk of malignant transformation, are confusing if AK is regarded as established squamous carcinoma. Whichever of these approaches is correct there is no doubt that AK is a strong predictor of basal cell carcinoma (BCC) and SCC and its presence therefore helps to identify those at risk who need advice and observation.

Aetiology and epidemiology

Actinic keratoses have long been recognized as a consequence of cumulative long-term sun exposure. In addition AKs can develop as a result of ultraviolet light exposure from artificial sources used in therapy (UVB and PUVA) or even from sun beds. Their distribution on the body reflects the intensity of sun exposure with the greatest number being found on the head, neck, forearm and hands. The prevalence of AKs rises with increasing age and exposure to ultraviolet light and with an ageing population more people are likely to develop these premalignant lesions. Men are more often affected than women, particularly at a younger age – this may reflect occupational ultraviolet light exposure.

The aetiology is not only environmental for host factors, in particular genetic influences play an important part. Firstly, individuals with fair skin, blue eyes and blond hair are more prone to developing actinic keratoses than those with darker skins. Indeed in black-skinned races these keratoses are rare. Secondly there are a number of syndromes which predispose those affected to ultraviolet damage as a result of defective melanin or DNA. Examples are albinism, xeroderma pigmentosum and Bloom's syndrome. In these groups AK may be seen as early as 8 years of age. These rare diseases are also discussed in Chapters 3–5.

Human studies suggest that oncogenes together with ultraviolet light and other factors affect the induction of AKs and their progression to SCC. Aberrations of the p53 tumour suppresser gene can be found in 90% of SCCs and they are also present in AKs. Clonal expansion of p53 mutated cells has been demonstrated in sunburn reactions.

Accurate data on the prevalence of AK is difficult to obtain. Most studies look at selected groups such as those attending hospital. Diagnostic accuracy is a further problem with inexperienced observers, and in no study has histological confirmation been available. One study in Ireland found an 11% prevalence rate in adults over the age of 21 and in Australia a study of 20–69 year olds found a rate of 40%.

Natural history

Some AKs will disappear spontaneously or after sun avoidance. Studies of this phenomenon are difficult to pursue as a histological diagnosis cannot be made at the outset. In one study of people with multiple keratoses followed over a 12-month period 36% had spontaneous remission of at least one lesion and there was an overall remission rate of 10%.

Some AKs remain unchanged and others will progress and develop into SCC. The risk of malignant transformation is low in any individual AK (estimated at < 1% per annum) but in patients with numerous lesions over a 10-year period, the risk of developing SCC has been estimated at around 10%. This risk is greatly increased by continued sun exposure or concurrent immunosuppression as seen for example in organ transplant recipients.

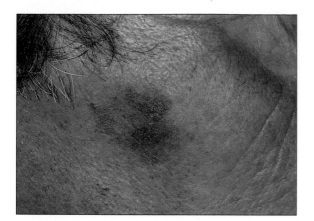

Figure 2.1
Early actinic keratosis with marked
telangiectasia.

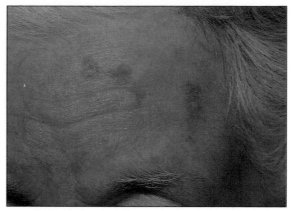

Figure 2.2
Several small keratoses.

Clinical features

The earliest evidence of AK is a tiny red telangiectatic spot, which passes unnoticed until
the diagnostic dry, rough, adherent scaling
appears. The telangiectatic appearance may
persist as it grows, producing little or no scale
(Figure 2.1). More often mild hyperkeratosis
covers most of the patch producing a lesion
which can be skin coloured to red but may
appear yellow or brown (Figure 2.2). The scale
is firmly attached and can only be picked off
with difficulty revealing bleeding points. The
lesions are clearly demarcated (Figure 2.3),
round or irregular in shape and usually
between 3 and 6 mm in diameter but occasionally several centimetres across (Figure 2.4).
Sometimes small lesions are more easily felt
than visualized. Actinic keratoses may be
solitary but are usually multiple and may
coalesce into plaques or sheets. On the head
and neck the common pattern is flat but they
may develop a thick, heaped-up, yellow crust
which on the undersurface is exudative; this

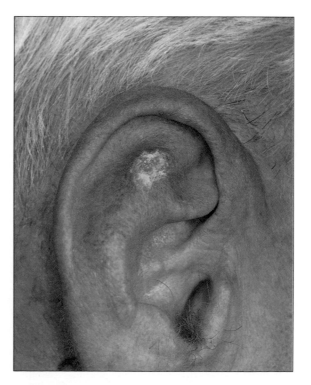

Figure 2.3
Well-defined keratosis with firmly adherent
surface.

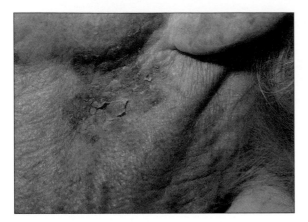

Figure 2.4
Large lesion with loose, yellow keratin.
Marked sun damage in adjacent skin.

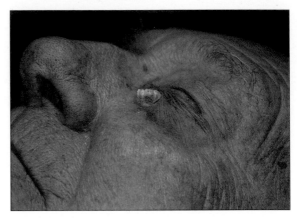

Figure 2.6
Actinic keratosis producing a cutaneous
horn.

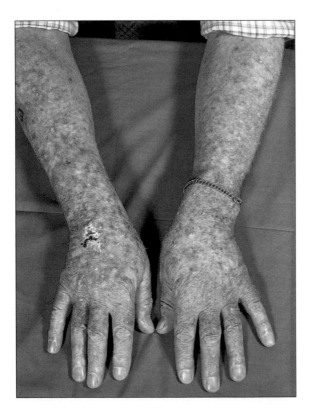

Figure 2.5
Extensive, hypertrophic keratoses on
forearms and hands.

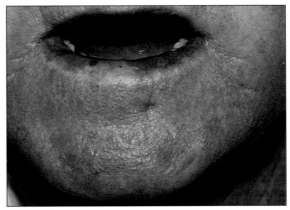

Figure 2.7
Actinic cheilitis with loss of the distinct
vermilion border.

can be lifted off revealing a glistening red
surface.

Lesions tend to be thicker on the back of the
hands and on the forearms (Figure 2.5).
Hyperkeratotic lesions in this area have a
higher rate of malignant transformation. At
any site an AK may produce a compact

cutaneous horn (Figure 2.6) and up to 15% of these have a malignant base. Generally actinic keratoses are asymptomatic but occasionally patients report irritation or a tingling sensation in sunlight.

Actinic change on the lips is known as actinic cheilitis and appears usually on the lower lip as a diffuse scaling with focal hyperkeratosis (Figure 2.7). Symptoms are peeling, irritation and pain. Ulceration, vertical fissures and loss of a sharp vermilion border may indicate malignant change and at this site metastasis is much more likely.

Other evidence of sun damage is usually evident in patients with AKs. Solar elastosis with coarse, yellowish, wrinkled skin and solar lentigines may be seen.

Differential diagnosis

Diagnosis of AK is usually straightforward. The two chief differential diagnoses are squamous carcinoma and other unrelated disorders. The previous section has highlighted the increased risk of malignancy in some clinical types of AK and there should be a low threshold for biopsy in these types.

Seborrhoeic keratoses can cause diagnostic problems appearing as lightly pigmented scaly patches, cutaneous horns or inflamed, weeping, hypertrophic lesions. It should also be remembered that keratoses due to ionizing and infrared radiation, tar and arsenic may look similar although the distribution is likely to vary. Bowen's disease and BCC may have a very similar appearance and distribution to AK. Frequently the conditions will coexist making it difficult to identify multiple lesions accurately.

At times inflammatory skin diseases come into the differential diagnosis. Small patches of eczema and psoriasis may persist and if present in sun-exposed sites can cause difficulties. Some elderly balding men develop scaly seborrhoeic eczema in the same area as their actinic damage. Discoid lupus erythematosus is usually redder in colour with a detachable scale and follicular plugging but it often occurs in the same distribution as AK on the face.

Pathology

As discussed in the introduction to this chapter there are two views about the status of AK – premalignant or malignant. Here the premalignant designation is used. Actinic keratosis is a cutaneous dysplasia confined to the epidermis. Epidermal cells are abnormal, appearing paler and variable in size and shape with nuclear atypia. Some nuclei are enlarged and contain prominent nucleoli. Other keratinocytes may be multinucleated or vacuolated with occasional mitotic figures. The epidermal cells have a paler cytoplasm and mature through an absent or diminished granular layer to form a parakeratotic scale of varying thickness. There is usually some irregular acanthosis and more dysplastic lesions show epidermal hypertrophy with hyperkeratosis and parakeratosis. The boundary between affected and normal epidermis is distinct. The affected zone tends to grow under the normal epidermis and may separate from it by a cleft – the so-called acantholytic keratosis.

If the dysplastic keratinocytes replace the entire epidermis the lesion is designated as a Bowenoid variant. Progression to invasive SCC is indicated by acanthosis with budding proliferation of keratinocytes from the lower epidermis penetrating into the dermis and associated capillary proliferation. Histology of cutaneous SCC often shows a link with contiguous AK.

Management

Prevention

The reduction of sunlight exposure in children may substantially decrease the incidence of AK and SCC later in life. Even in patients with established AKs, sun avoidance and regular use of sunscreens will help to reduce the incidence of new lesions and prevent malignant transformation. Organ transplant recipients on immunosuppression and other patients who are immunosuppressed are at greater risk of developing AKs and also of malignant transformation to SCC. One study has suggested that a low-fat diet may reduce the rate of development of AK but this requires confirmation.

Treatment (for details of techniques see Chapter 7)

A variety of treatments are available for AKs. There may be a place for observation of single or multiple lesions and some very elderly people may positively refuse any intervention. For those individuals with multiple lesions the policy is normally of control and observation rather than eradication of every lesion at the earliest opportunity. Usually a combination of different modalities including cryotherapy, curettage and 5-fluorouracil (5-FU) is sufficient.

Cryotherapy: Superficial AKs are most easily removed by rapid freezing with liquid nitrogen using a single freeze–thaw cycle of 5–10 s. This heals with scabbing in a week or 10 days and usually gives an excellent cosmetic result without scarring. Cryotherapy can be used close to the eyes, even on the eyelids, but may produce considerable swelling, particularly in elderly skin, so patients must be warned. Lesions which have undergone cryotherapy on elderly lower legs are often very slow to heal and may ulcerate so other modalities may be better at this site. Cryotherapy is uncomfortable so if there are multiple lesions treatment may have to be staggered. Some clinicians recommend application of a very potent topical steroid ointment to the lesion immediately after cryosurgery to reduce the inflammatory reaction. Nonsteroidal anti-inflammatory drugs may help reduce pain if severe.

Surgery: Destruction by curettage and cautery or electrodesiccation is also effective though more time consuming (and expensive) and it is more likely to leave superficial scarring. If the AK is thicker or there is doubt as to the diagnosis, this method will yield tissue for histological examination. Full-thickness excision of AK is rarely performed by dermatologists (though more often by plastic surgeons, general surgeons and GPs) but it may be indicated if early invasive SCC is suspected. Formal excision allows proper interpretation of the histology – it is difficult to assess invasion from curetted specimens.

Topical agents: For patients with multiple lesions topical 5% 5-fluorouracil (5-FU) cream (Efudix) is very effective. The cream must be applied for 1–4 weeks and produces a brisk and severe inflammatory reaction with erosion of the keratoses and often some of the surrounding area, which may represent unsuspected disease. Normal skin is unaffected by the cream. As the reaction settles over 2 or 3 weeks the diffuse keratoses clear. Another topical treatment that may be helpful in diffuse AKs is tretinoin 0.025% (Retin A).

Chemical peels with trichloracetic acid, phenol or alpha-hydroxy acids may be helpful. Dermabrasion and carbon dioxide resurfacing laser have also been used in the treatment of extensive AKs but these are much more expensive modalities.

Bowen's disease

Introduction

In 1912 John Bowen, then Professor of Dermatology at Harvard Medical School, described skin lesions in two patients as 'chronic atypical epithelial proliferation'. In 1914 Jean Darier in Paris wrote to Bowen about his experience with two patients he recognized as having the same condition and suggested that Bowen's name be attached to the disease. Darier referred to this condition in his textbook as 'precancerous dermatosis of Bowen or dyskeratosis lenticularis et discoides'. This intra-epidermal SCC (carcinoma in situ) has since come to be known simply as 'Bowen's disease'.

Aetiology and epidemiology

Trauma, chemical carcinogens and radiation have been described as possible aetiological factors in the pathogenesis of BD. The most important chemical carcinogens are the inorganic arsenicals. These were, at one time, present in some herbal remedies and medications used in the treatment of psoriasis, eczema, lichen planus, lupus, syphilis and asthma. Exposure to arsenicals is possible in many forms including pesticides, weed killers and fungicides.

Bowen's disease occurs predominantly in the elderly and is most commonly diagnosed in the sixth to eighth decades. In the UK 80% of cases are in women[1] and the majority have lesions on the lower limb.[2] Other commonly affected areas are sun-exposed sites on the head and neck. This age distribution and sun-exposed distribution of BD implicates chronic ultraviolet exposure as a major aetiological factor. Bowen's disease is rare in black-skinned races and then usually affects non sun-exposed sites. Another aetiological agent is the human papilloma virus (HPV) which has been detected in lesions of BD. HPV16 has been especially implicated in carcinogenesis and is found in up to 30% of anogenital lesions.

A relationship between BD and internal malignancy was first reported in 1959 and seemed to be supported by subsequent studies. However a meta-analysis of 12 studies in 1989 failed to demonstrate a significant association.[3] Routine investigation for internal malignancy in patients with BD is therefore not justified.

Natural history

Unlike AK there is little to suggest that BD ever undergoes natural regression. Lesions tend to persist and grow slowly over many years eventually reaching sizes of 10 cm or more. The risk of progression to squamous carcinoma is hard to assess. Rates of up to 20% have been proposed but without sound backing. Only retrospective studies have been conducted and they suggest a rate of about 3%. The data in these studies dates from 15 to 40 years ago and at that time a greater proportion of BD may have been due to arsenic exposure; this makes it difficult to extrapolate the results to the present day. Bowen's disease on mucosal surfaces has a higher rate of malignant change.

Clinical features

Bowen's disease may occur anywhere on the skin or mucosal surfaces. On the skin the earliest change is a red patch with a variable amount of scale (Figure 2.8). There is gradual,

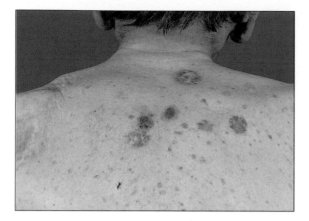

Figure 2.8
Early lesions appear as a red patch with a scaly surface as seen here in a patient with multiple lesions occurring years after radiotherapy.

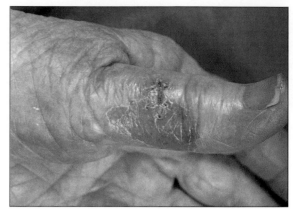

Figure 2.9
Lesion with a well-defined edge.

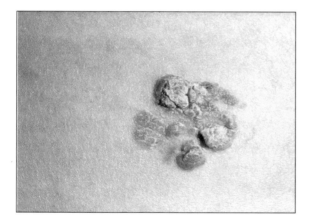

Figure 2.10
Hyperkeratosis and a scalloped edge.

radial growth, usually remaining fairly well demarcated (Figure 2.9) and often with a slightly scalloped edge. The scale is white or yellow and pieces can be detached leaving a moist surface. Hyperkeratosis may occur but is not site dependent (Figure 2.10). Occasionally there may be some pigmentation. Lesions

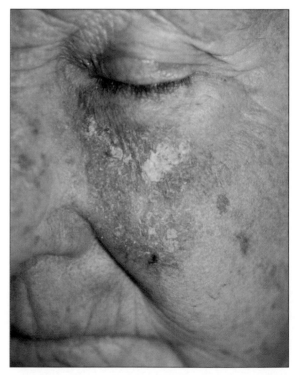

Figure 2.11
Large lesion > 4 cm on the cheek.

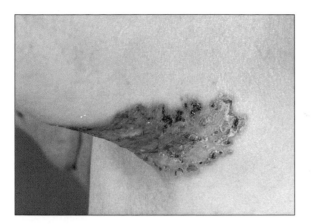

Figure 2.12
The surface may ulcerate.

range in size from a couple of millimetres to several centimetres (Figure 2.11) and are usually asymptomatic but may itch, ulcerate (Figure 2.12) and bleed (Figure 2.13). Bowen's disease usually occurs as a solitary lesion but may be multiple in up to 20% of patients. Lesions of BD may also occur on the conjunctiva, oral mucosa, perineum and nailbed (Figure 2.14).

In certain sites BD has an altered clinical appearance. On the palm it may ulcerate early, around the nailfolds it may appear as a viral

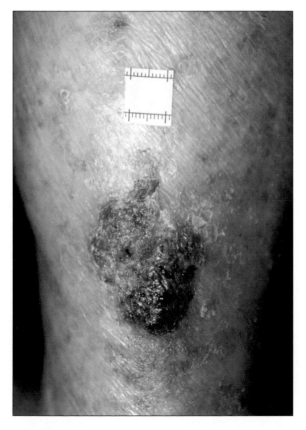

Figure 2.13
Bleeding lesion on the lower leg.

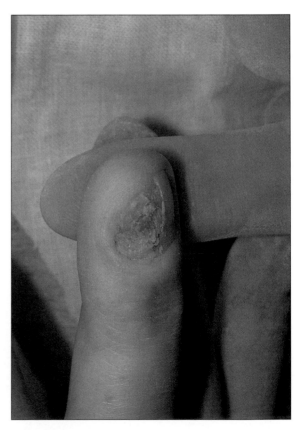

Figure 2.14
Bowen's disease may have some similarity to a viral wart around the nailbed.

wart with cracking and bleeding and on the eyelids it may resemble a wart. On the glans of the penis it has a bright red glistening surface. At this site it is seen almost exclusively in uncircumcised men and is referred to as erythroplasia of Queyrat.

Differential diagnosis

Even in the simple clinical setting of an elderly female with a solitary scaly patch on the lower leg present for 2 or more years there can be diagnostic problems. It has been shown that at this site experienced clinicians can easily confuse BD with BCC. When a sun-damaged individual has numerous red scaly lesions on the head, neck and lower limbs it is almost certain that some will be BD but others will be AKs or BCC and differentiation can be difficult. It is more important to distinguish BD from SCC: hyperkeratotic and ulcerated lesions can be particularly difficult.

The differential diagnosis includes eczema but in the discoid form this is often infected. Lichen simplex is often a solitary lesion but the surface cannot readily be detached. Psoriasis can be a particular problem as a few scaly lesions on the lower legs are a common presentation. Searching for other evidence of psoriasis is helpful and use of antipsoriatic creams may be effective as a therapeutic trial. Simple wart virus infections may show similar changes but when pared down will often reveal pinpoint bleeding or capillary thrombosis.

Rarely, lesions of BD may be pigmented and this can cause clinical confusion with other pigmented lesions such as seborrhoeic warts, lentigo or verrucous malignant melanoma. Bowenoid papulosis is usually seen on genital skin, is related to viral infection and though it may affect large areas it only rarely becomes malignant.

Pathology

Pathologically BD is an intra-epidermal SCC. The epidermis shows acanthosis with elongation of the rete ridges with atypical squamous cells proliferating through its entire thickness giving a disordered 'windblown' appearance. Many cells are highly atypical with large, hyperchromatic nuclei. The border between the epidermis and dermis however appears sharp and the basement membrane remains intact. Atypical cells in BD may extend into the follicular infundibula and cause replacement of the follicular epithelium down to the entrance of the sebaceous duct. This downward extension is thought to be the source of recurrence following superficial treatment methods.

Management
(see British Association of Dermatologists guidelines – Appendix I)

Prevention

Restricting ultraviolet exposure is presumed to be the most effective method although there are no studies to quantify this approach.

Treatment (for details of techniques see Chapters 7 and 8)

There may be a strong case for observation, rather than intervention, particularly in the elderly. If the appearances suggest BD and there are no symptoms there is little to be gained by treatment. The chief aim of therapy is to relieve symptoms or prevent a serious outcome. If the lesion is small, thin, slowly progressive and in an area where poor healing may be expected then observation is probably the right approach.

A number of factors need to be considered when deciding on the management of BD. Usually the diagnosis is clinical but if there is doubt or concern about the presence of invasive SCC then a biopsy should be taken. It is best to sample the thickest part of the lesion or that part which has ulcerated. Failure of part of a lesion to respond to treatment should suggest the need for a biopsy in case there is an area of malignant change.

A number of modalities are available for the treatment of BD. The treatment should be chosen on the basis of efficacy, low recurrence rates, patient acceptability and low risk of side effects and complications. There is an overall recurrence rate of more than 20% and this is probably related to poorly defined margins and follicular involvement.

Surgery

Surgical excision is often recommended because it enables removal of the abnormal area to a depth that includes the skin appendages, which are considered to be the main source of recurrence. Pathological examination of the excised specimen also allows more detailed exclusion of invasive SCC and gives some indication of complete excision. However surgery is not the most common treatment used because other modalities, such as cryotherapy, are quicker and easier and can be done in an outpatient setting. Surgery may require complex repairs such as grafts, there may be healing problems in some areas and at some sites, for example the penis, it can be mutilating.

Cryosurgery

Cryosurgery is popular because of its simplicity. The range of protocols used in different studies makes comparison difficult but the most successful treatments were either a single 30-s freeze–thaw cycle or two 20-s cycles. Overall they give a recurrence rate of less than 10% at 1 year. It is uncomfortable especially when multiple lesions are treated. Healing is another important consideration, especially as so many Bowen's patches are on the lower leg. Some experts warn against large doses of cryotherapy for this reason. However in one study aggressive cryosurgery (two 20-s freezes) was compared to radiotherapy and healing was superior in the freezing group.

Topical 5-fluorouracil

This is widely used in different concentrations but the currently available formulation in the UK is 5%. Topical 5-FU requires an extended treatment period and can produce significant inflammation and discomfort, but may be helpful for multiple lesions.

Photodynamic therapy

Photodynamic therapy offers excellent healing with a very good cosmetic result so that in the few centres that it is available it is often considered the treatment of choice for BD on the lower legs of elderly patients.

Curettage and cautery, shave excision, laser ablation and radiotherapy

Curettage and shave excision are simple techniques but will not give higher cure rates than excision. In a recent study using a disposable ring curette compared to cryosurgery the curettage was associated with lower recurrence rates and shorter healing times, less pain and fewer complications. Laser ablation is another superficial treatment but there are few data available. Radiotherapy has given excellent cure rates but it is time consuming and poor healing, especially on the lower leg, was a problem in 20% of patients.

Site-specific treatment

- *Digits:* Excision is often used especially around the nail unit. Micrographic surgery has the advantage of being tissue sparing.
- *Genitals:* The risk of invasive change is greater than at other sites and a more aggressive approach is necessary. There are no big studies but cryosurgery, carbon dioxide laser surgery, 5-FU and micrographic surgery have all been used with success. Perianal BD should also be treated energetically. Even wide excision has a recurrence rate of 30%. Radiotherapy may have a place for large or recurrent lesions.

Treatment failure and relapse

This is often attributed to the extension of disease down the hair follicles and indeed the recurrence often appears as dotted areas in the centre of the treated patch. Recurrence at the margins may be due to difficulty visualizing the extent of the disease. It may be that the relatively indolent behaviour of this disease and its occurrence on difficult sites like the lower leg lead the clinician to use narrower margins of excision than are needed.

Follow-up policy

Follow-up serves two functions. The first is to assess the success of the treatment and this is appropriate between 3 and 6 months. The second is to screen for further lesions of BD and other skin tumours. The need will depend on the patient's general state of health, reliability in terms of self-examination and the interest and skill of their GP who may be able to take over this role.

Lentigo maligna

Introduction

Lentigo maligna is an in-situ pattern of malignant melanoma. One of the earliest descriptions of it was in 1892 and it is still sometimes referred to by the author's name – Hutchinson's freckle. In the early stages it is hard to differentiate clinically from other pigmented lesions such as solar lentigo and flat seborrhoeic warts and it may be equally hard to distinguish histologically from solar lentigo in severely photodamaged skin. For these reasons LM often reaches a large size before the diagnosis is made. There has also been a poor understanding of its natural history and the risk of malignant change. Once malignant change has taken place the metastatic potential of this tumour is the same as for malignant melanoma elsewhere.

Aetiology and epidemiology

This is poorly understood but sunlight plays a part as many cases occur on sun-exposed sites. It is however found in other sites where the trigger factors are unknown.

Natural history

The rate of growth seems to be highly variable but it is unlikely that growth ever ceases. In a number of cases dermal invasion is seen and it is then called a lentigo maligna melanoma (LMM). Estimates of the frequency of malig-

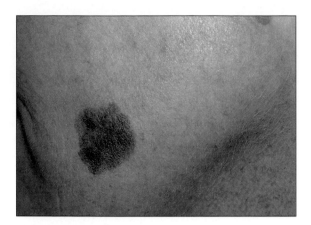

Figure 2.15
Variation in pigmentation with slightly irregular edge.

nant change vary from 5 to 50%. One study estimated that 1% of LM per year transform in patients over 45 years of age. Head and neck lesions account for 90% of those which become malignant. At one time it was believed that LMM had a better prognosis than other melanomas but it is now clear that after acccounting for Breslow thickness and site the prognosis for LMM is the same.

Clinical features

Lentigo maligna begins as a flat, pigmented lesion; usually it is seen on sun-exposed skin of the head and neck, however almost any area may be affected and it is important not to exclude the diagnosis on clinical grounds simply because of an unusual location. It can be uniform in colour at the outset making it difficult to diagnose but with time both the colour and border become more irregular (Figure 2.15). Early lesions may be light brown or dark but with time darker pigmentation is often seen. The growth may be very

slow taking years to achieve the size of 2 cm; however the lesion will continue to grow inexorably and may eventually grow to about 10 cm. Amelanotic LM may be very difficult to diagnose when it appears as an erythematous patch. It can arise de novo or develop from a previously pigmented lesion. This situation may also be seen following inadequate cryosurgical treatment of LM.

Differential diagnosis

Actinically damaged skin may contain a variety of pigmented changes making accurate diagnosis difficult. Solar elastosis usually has a yellow/brown colour and poorly defined edges. Actinic lentigo (simple or senile lentigo) usually has a uniform colour and fairly even edges, ranging from a few millimetres to a centimetre in diameter. The most common sites are the face and the dorsum of the hand. Their number tends to increase with age so that in elderly people almost everybody will have one or more actinic lentigo. Flat, early seborrhoeic warts may resemble LM and require incisional biopsy to distinguish them (Figure 2.16). Areas of an LM may develop invasive melanoma either as a nodule or a thickened patch (Figure 2.17) and this should trigger rapid therapeutic intervention. The rare amelanotic form of LM may resemble an inflammatory dermatosis, BD or the telangiectatic variant of solar keratosis. The commonest presentation is on the face of older women.

Dermatoscopy with × 10 magnification can help to distinguish between LM, simple lentigo and early seborrhoeic keratosis. In one study[4] of 87 patients presenting with 37 malignant and 50 benign pigmented skin lesions on the face, dermatoscopy gave a high rate of diagnostic accuracy. The most important factors were asymmetrical pigmented follicular openings, dark rhomboid structures, slate

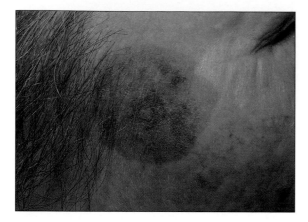

Figure 2.16
Flat seborrhoeic warts may resemble lentigo
maligna.

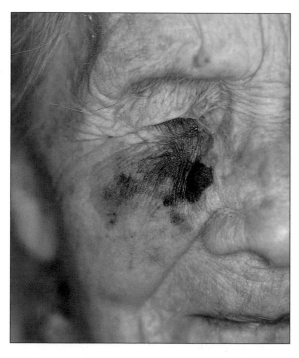

Figure 2.17
A long-standing lentigo maligna developed
darkening and thickening medially and this
represented development of invasive
melanoma.

grey globules and slate grey dots. Dermato-
scopic features on the face differed from
criteria used in other locations.

Pathology

There is a proliferation of pigmented dendritic
melanocytes in a lentiginous arrangement with
or without nests. There is usually a varying
degree of nuclear atypia within an atrophic
epidermis. In early lesions and at the periphery
of established lesions there may be great difficulty differentiating between the atypical
melanocytes of LM and the pleomorphic
atypical melanocytes in skin subjected to long-
term sun exposure.

Some dermatologists consider LM to be an
atypical melanocytic hyperplasia while others
believe it is melanoma in situ. It has been
suggested[5] that there are indeed two subsets
with some lesions showing features purely of
hyperplasia while others have additional
features: individual and nests of cells throughout the epidermis, confluence of the
melanocytes replacing the basal region, uniformity of the cytological atypia and nesting of
uniformly atypical melanocytes. The authors
felt that the second group represented
melanoma in situ and that they may be more
aggressive lesions. Furthermore they examined
the intra-epidermal component of malignant
melanoma (LMM type) and found that they
shared the same features that they had previously identified for the in-situ melanoma type
of LM.

Management

Surgery

Most experts agree that melanoma of the in-
situ variety should be cured in all cases when

removed with a 2–5 mm margin. In theory this should also apply to the LM variants of in-situ melanoma. However using these margins has led to recurrence rates of up to 10% and for larger lesions the rates may be even higher. It has been suggested that using a Wood's light to delineate the clinical margins gives improved results. The reason for recurrence is presumably due to subclinical extension of abnormal cells. It has already been mentioned in the discussion of pathology that interpreting melanocytic atypia can be difficult. So although micrographic surgery may give the highest cure rate there are still some recurrences. The reason for this may be the difficulty in interpreting melanocytic atypia on frozen sections. Paraffin-embedded sections are often employed but even so the atypical cells of lentiginous proliferation may look similar to the atypical melanocytes seen in chronically sun-damaged skin.

The concept of removing the lesion and leaving the wound open and awaiting interpretation of the paraffin-embedded sections is appealing. Not only may further peripheral excision be required but also in up to 20% of cases there may be evidence of invasive melanoma somewhere in the lesion that was not clinically obvious. If this is found the clinician may then be inclined to take a still wider margin.

Nonsurgical methods

It is important to take several biopsies depending on the size of the lesion. If a nonsurgical method is to be used the clinician needs to be as certain as possible that there is no invasive melanoma present.

Radiotherapy

In one study involving 42 patients with LM followed for a mean of 2 years, fractionated radiotherapy was effective in all case with no recurrences noted. In some of the studies pretreatment biopsies were not taken. It is impossible to assess whether failure of treatment, leading later to excision and the discovery of invasive melanoma, represents true failure of the original method or simply failure to recognize that an invasive component was present before treatment. Several studies give approximately the same cure rate of 90–93%. Cosmetic results may be poor in up to 10% of patients.

Cryosurgery (for details of techniques see Chapter 7)

In theory this should be an excellent treatment because melanocytes are very sensitive to cold. The growth of LM down the follicular epithelium means that some of the abnormal melanocytes may be up to 3 mm deep and it is essential to get effective cell death at this depth. The total freeze time in reported studies is usually between 45 and 60 s with a lateral freeze of approximately 1 cm. Using the spot-freeze method (Chapter 7) a double 20-s freeze–thaw cycle is often used. These doses will inevitably lead to slow healing over 6–12 weeks but the cosmetic results tend to be good.

Other methods

Laser therapy is still at an experimental stage. There are theoretical advantages for such treatments because of the small upset to the patient. The neodymium yag laser has been used with success in a few cases whereas the Q Switched Ruby laser reportedly failed in two atypical lentigo. Curettage and cautery, 5-FU, azeleic acid and retinoic acid have all been used but there is no good evidence to suggest that any of these methods have a place in routine clinical practice.

In a review of all the available therapies for LM[6] the authors concluded that micrographic surgery has the highest cure rate and conventional surgery, cryosurgery and radiotherapy all have recurrence rates in the order of 7–10%. On the basis of the available literature, all three of these treatments could be recommended as primary treatments for LM. The authors also stress the importance of the treating physician being skilled in the appropriate modality.

References

1. Ball SB, Dawber RP (1998) Treatment of cutaneous Bowen's disease with particular emphasis on the problem of lower leg lesions, *Australas J Dermatol* **39**:63–70.
2. Cox NH (1994) Body site distribution of Bowen's disease, *Br J Dermatol* **130**:714–16.
3. Lycka BA (1989) Bowen's disease and internal malignancy: A meta-analysis, *Int J Dermatol* **28**:531–3.
4. Schiffner R, Schiffner-Rohe J, Vogt T et al (2000) Improvement of early recognition of lentigo maligna using dermatoscopy, *J Am Acad Dermatol* **42**:25–32.
5. Flotte TJ, Mihm MC (1999) Lentigo maligna and malignant melanoma in situ, lentigo maligna type, *Human Pathol* **30**:533–6.
6. Gaspar ZS, Dawber RPR (1997) Treatment of lentigo maligna, *Australas J Dermatol* **38**:1–6.

Bibliography

Schwartz RA (1997) The actinic keratosis, *CME Dermatol Surg* **23**:1009–19.

Frost CA, Green AC (1994) Epidemiology of solar keratoses, *Br J Dermatol* **131**:455–64.

Callen JP, Bickers DR, Moy RL (1997) Actinic keratoses, *J Am Acad Dermatol* **30**:650–3.

Ragi G, Turner MS, Klein LE, Stoll HL (1998) Pigmented Bowen's disease and review of 420 Bowen's disease lesions, *J Derm Surg Oncol* **14**:765–9.

Kossard S, Rosen R (1992) Cutaneous Bowen's disease. An analysis of 1001 cases according to age, sex, and site, *J Am Acad Dermatol* **27**:406–10.

Cohen LM (1995) Lentigo maligna and lentigo maligna melanoma, *J Am Acad Dermatol* **33**:923–36.

3 Basal cell carcinoma

Introduction

Basal cell carcinoma (BCC) is the most common cancer affecting humans. It arises almost exclusively in hair-bearing skin, usually in sun-damaged, fair people over 50 years old and metastasizes only extremely rarely. It has a wide range of clinical appearances, yet is usually easy to diagnose. Probably the first description of this tumour was in 1712 and the next was in Jacob's report from Dublin, Ireland in 1827: the long interval perhaps emphasizes how rare it used to be. Because it is relatively benign in most cases, it is often dismissed as being unimportant, but the consequence of incorrect treatment and management can be disfiguring and life threatening.

Aetiology and epidemiology

The most important risk factor for BCC is solar ultraviolet radiation.[1] Perhaps it is no coincidence that the earliest reports of BCC are in Anglo-Saxons or Celts, as many surveys have found that those with Type I skin with red/blond hair and blue/green eyes are most susceptible. Basal cell carcinoma shows more similarity to melanoma, in its relationship to solar irradiation, than it does to squamous cell carcinoma (SCC). Episodes of painful sunburn and probably early life exposure are important. The cumulative effect of UVB may be less crucial than it is with SCC. Depletion of the ozone layer increases the amount of ultraviolet radiation to which we are all exposed but it has a smaller effect than the changes in lifestyle which have occurred over the last 25 years. The mechanism of injury by ultraviolet radiation is complex. There is direct damage to DNA, the repair mechanisms, the immune system and mutations in p53 suppresser genes.

Rising incidence

There is well-publicized evidence that the incidence of all types of skin cancer is rising worldwide. Because cancer registries do not all record BCC and none record multiple tumours in one individual, it is difficult to compare data widely. However there has been careful documentation in some areas. In North Humberside[2] the age-standardized incidence of BCC per 100 000 population in 1978 was 38 among men and 37 among women. For 1991 the corresponding figures were 115 and 103 for men and women. This represented an increase of 14% and 12% for men and women respectively. In a similar study conducted in Stockholm 10 years earlier, between 1971 and 1980, the increase was 14% for men and 10% for women.

Skin colour and ethnicity

The incidence in white-skinned races is approximately 70 times that in black-skinned races, and albino black-skinned people have a higher incidence than those with normal pigment, conclusively demonstrating the protective role of melanin. Rare though it is in black-skinned people, it still primarily occurs on sun-exposed skin. Ethnic origin is also important in white-skinned populations so that southern Europeans have a lower incidence than northern Europeans. In children the presence of freckling on the arms is a predictor of increased susceptibility in later life and in another study more than 4 naevi > 5 mm diameter on the back was also an indicator.

Geography and ultraviolet radiation

Figures from around the world repeatedly demonstrate a rise in the incidence of skin cancer. Some of this may be due to more efficient registration and an ageing population with increased sun exposure, but the rise is consistent everywhere at between 3–7% per year. Generally the incidence is greater in white-skinned races who live in closer proximity to the equator: in Iceland the annual incidence is 10 per 100 000 while in Western Australia figures of over 788 per 100 000 men are seen. Even in the UK the incidence increases from Scotland towards Cornwall, where the incidence is now over 300 per 100 000.

Therapeutic radiation and suntanning lamps

It has been shown that more than 10 exposures per year to tanning devices induces a significant risk to the development of BCC, SCC and malignant melanoma (MM). Equally the carcinogenic effect of PUVA in patients who require multiple repeated courses is recognized: the incidence of SCC rises much more than BCC.

Ionizing radiation was historically used therapeutically in a number of settings. An increased number of BCCs are now seen on the scalp in people who were treated for tinea capitis, over the spine at the site of treatment for ankylosing spondylitis and at the site of application of thorium X used to treat haemangiomas. These tumours appear after a lag period of 20–50 years. Claims for the safety of modern radiotherapy, when used for conditions such as keloid, may be premature.

Immunosuppression

Renal transplant patients have a huge increase in the incidence of SCC and to a lesser extent BCC. In a Dutch study it was 10 times higher than in the general population over a 20-year period. People suffering with various forms of leukaemia and lymphoma also have increased rates of nonmelanoma skin cancer (NMSC). The ratio of BCC:SCC is similar to that in the general population but the tumours are often more aggressive with a higher recurrence rate than expected. The situation is similar in people with AIDS.

Familial and congenital conditions

It is important to recognize individuals who have familial syndromes which put them at greater risk of developing multiple tumours. They require follow-up for new tumours and other manifestations and genetic counselling should be available. Some of these genetic disorders are predominantly associated with cutaneous tumours. In Gorlin's syndrome there are multiple BCCs, either naevoid or typical in appearance, and anomalies such as palmopalmar pits, dental cysts, rib and spine abnormalities. In Bazex syndrome follicular atrophoderma presents as ice-pick marks and enlarged follicular orifices on the dorsum of the hands, elbows, feet and face, sometimes with facial eczema, anhidrosis and hypotrichosis. Basal cell carcinomas resembling cellular naevi appear on the face from the second decade. Xeroderma pigmentosum is an autosomal recessive disorder giving extreme light sensitivity and a massively increased risk of skin cancer. Other syndromes that can include increased risk of BCC, are Muir–Torre, Cowden and albinism.

Lesions with malignant potential

Naevus sebaceous occurs in about 0.3% of neonates. It is usually present at birth, appearing on the head and neck, with a characteristic orange–yellow colour. There is a 5% risk of malignant transformation especially to BCC usually from teenage onwards. Excision around the time of puberty is advised. Syringocystadenoma papilliferum is another lesion at risk of developing BCC. Scars from trauma, surgery, burns and vaccination sites have all been reported as being sites of BCC formation.

Site distribution

At least 75% of first tumours are on the face but the distribution does not entirely correlate with the areas of greatest sun exposure. Basal cell carcinoma is common around the inner canthus and behind the ear, but rare on the dorsum of the hand or forearm. It is not infrequent on the lower back, and may even be seen on the vulva. Basal cell carcinoma on the lower leg is more common in women than men; if sunshine is relevant stockings seem to provide little protection.

Natural history

The description of rodent ulcer by Arthur Jacob, in Chapter 1, gives a graphic account of the slow inexorable progression of this tumour. However neglected tumours are still seen today sometimes extending over the entire scalp, destroying the eyelids or nasal tissues. It is the occasional sight of these horrific tumours that serves as a reminder that BCC must be taken seriously and assessed carefully on every occasion.

Equally, many BCCs grow so slowly that 20 years or so may elapse before the patient feels the need to consult their medical practitioner. In one study 31 patients with BCC had their tumour measured at diagnosis and again 2 months later just before surgery. Over this period some increased and others decreased in size but the changes did not reach statistical significance. The rate of progression of BCC depends on the histological type and host factors. In younger people tumours appear to be more difficult to eradicate.

Clinical features

Basal cell carcinomas may be divided, on clinical grounds, into six relatively distinct categories (Table 3.1) although there is often some overlap of features. Pigmentation of

Table 3.1
Types of basal cell carcinoma.

Nodulo-ulcerative, cystic
Superficial
Multifocal
Morphoeic
Bowenoid
Poorly differentiated

varying density may be seen in any of these types and overall in about 2%. In around 10% of cases more that one BCC may be present and occasionally five or more separate primary tumours may be found. Once a BCC has been diagnosed a thorough search should be made for others. Common sites which are often missed include the hairline, around the eyes (especially in spectacle wearers), behind the ears of men and on the lower legs of women.

Some types of tumour are more likely to appear at certain anatomical sites:

- head and neck – nodulo-ulcerative, cystic, multifocal, morphoeic,
- trunk – nodulo-ulcerative, cystic, super-ficial,
- lower limbs – Bowenoid.

Nodulo-ulcerative, cystic
(Figures 3.1 and 3.2)

This usually begins as a small pink semitranslucent ('pearly') papule which may have a depressed centre from an early stage. There is slow enlargement of the tumour, during which time the nodulo-ulcerative type will develop a marked depression in the centre presaging ulceration while the cystic type will maintain a more dome-shaped structure.

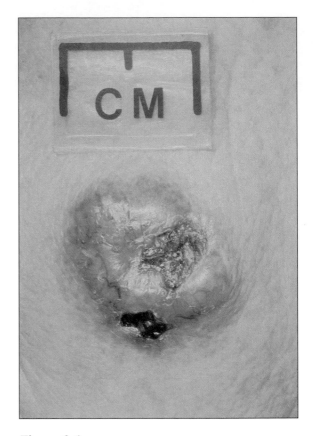

Figure 3.1
Nodulo-ulcerative basal cell carcinoma with incipient ulceration.

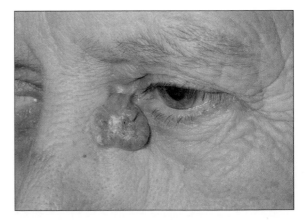

Figure 3.2
Cystic basal cell carcinoma.

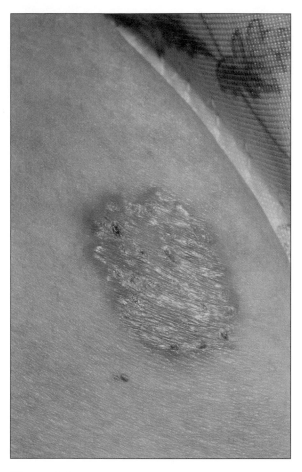

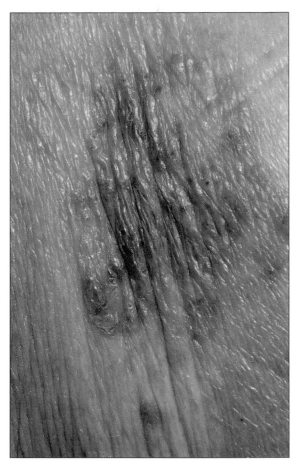

Figure 3.3
Superficial basal cell carcinoma (rolled edge clearly apparent).

Figure 3.4
Superficial basal cell carcinoma.

Telangiectasia, usually seen traversing the raised ('rolled') edge in a radial fashion becomes more apparent as the tumour grows.

Superficial (Figures 3.3 and 3.4)

Superficial BCCs are usually found on the trunk and may be multiple especially years after radiotherapy to the area. The lesions appear as flat, red patches and when small may be difficult to identify as a BCC. However even in small lesions the typical beaded edge of a BCC may be visible. In large, well-developed tumours the rolled edge is often incomplete. As they enlarge the surface becomes more fragile and focal areas of scale, crust and blood clot may appear. If neglected these can achieve very large sizes but they remain true to type and therefore superficial.

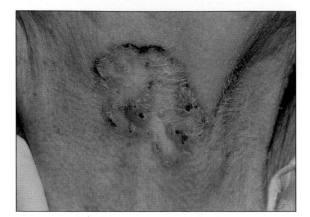

Figure 3.5
Multifocal basal cell carcinoma showing
areas of regression.

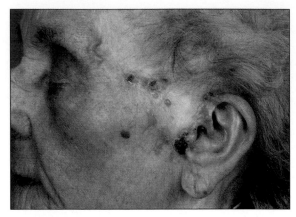

Figure 3.6
Multifocal basal cell carcinoma on temple
and hair-bearing scalp.

Multifocal (Figures 3.5 and 3.6)

These are most common on the head and neck.
The name is acquired from the histological
appearances of apparently isolated nodules of
BCC. In practice they are contiguous, with
fine strands of tumour cells connecting the
nodules. The nodules of the tumour are largely
confined to the upper dermis and epidermis.

Multifocal BCC starts as a pale nodule and
expands outwards with areas of apparent
regression developing between the nodules. The
edge is well-defined and usually continuous
around the tumour margin. Scale, crust and
blood clot may occur but they are paler than in
the superficial type. Large tumours are common
as they often remain unrecognized. Multiple
lesions may be seen especially on the scalp.

Morphoeic and infiltrative
(Figures 3.7 and 3.8)

Many BCCs show some sclerotic features and
may show an infiltrative pattern histologically.

However a true morphoeic BCC is mono-
morphic, white or waxy. Not uncommonly it
presents as a spontaneous 'scar' or pit and is
seen almost exclusively on the face. The
margins are usually much wider than is clinically apparent and recurrence is more common
after surgical excision. It has a greater tendency
to track down embryonic fusion planes and
along neurovascular bundles.

Bowenoid (Figures 3.9 and 3.10)

This type is usually found on the lower legs
of women with sun-damaged skin. There is
usually scale present and an absence of the
usual BCC features such as telangiectasia and
a rolled edge. Clinically it most closely resembles either a patch of Bowen's disease (BD) or
a Bowenoid keratosis. The diagnosis is usually
made histologically.

Poorly differentiated (Figure 3.11)

These are covered with a thick crust with
granulation tissue underneath. On clinical

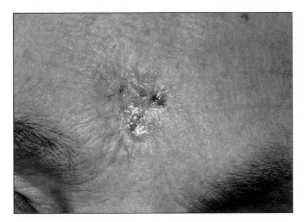

Figure 3.7
Morphoeic basal cell carcinoma with central
ulceration.

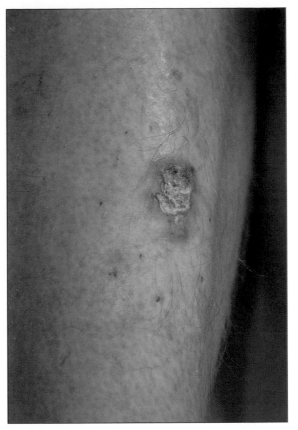

Figure 3.9
Bowenoid basal cell carcinoma on lower leg.

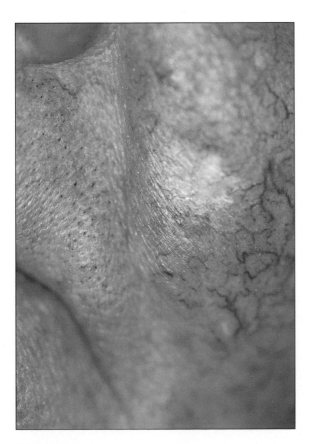

Figure 3.8
Solid morphoeic basal cell carcinoma.

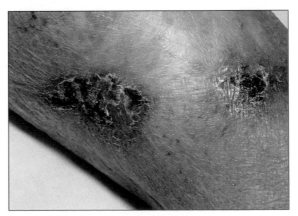

Figure 3.10
Bowenoid basal cell carcinoma.

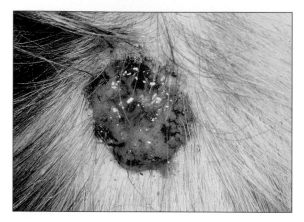

Figure 3.11
Poorly differentiated basal cell carcinoma.

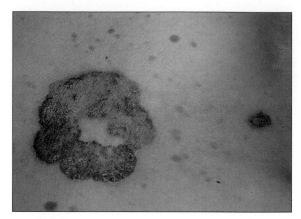

Figure 3.12
Pigmented basal cell carcinoma.

grounds they cannot be easily distinguished from other poorly differentiated tumours.

Other clinical variants

Unusual variants include the naevoid lesions seen in Gorlin's syndrome and keloidal and linear growth patterns. Pigmentation can be a feature of any form of BCC (Figures 3.12 and 3.13) and is discussed in the 'Pathology' section.

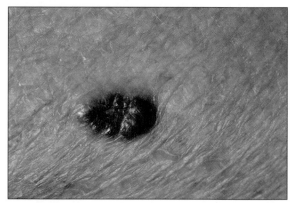

Figure 3.13
Pigmented basal cell carcinoma.

Extensive and neglected tumours

Basal cell carcinoma may become extensive for a variety of reasons. The tumour may not be obvious as in the case of a morphoeic lesion or it may frighten the patient who suppresses their awareness and hides it (Figure 3.14). It may have been misdiagnosed as a benign lesion or alternatively having been correctly diagnosed it may then have been inadequately or inappropriately treated by various modalities.

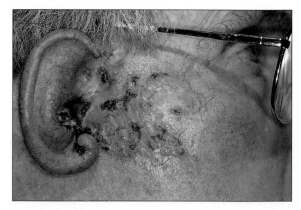

Figure 3.14
Neglected extensive tumour.

Sometimes the scarring associated with multiple treatments conceals the extent of the disease. The factors linked to recurrence are discussed in this chapter. Frequently the cause of large tumours is a combination of several events.

Metastases

Basal cell carcinomas rarely metastasize. Up to 1984 only 205 cases were reported in the literature giving an incidence of less than 0.01%. The most common site was the head and most were basi-squamous. Several contributing factors were identified. The tumours tended to be large and recurrent after several attempts at clearance. The site tended to facilitate easy spread, for example, spillover into an airway. Once metastasis has occurred the prognosis is poor with an average 1-year survival of 20%.

Death

There are few good data on mortality from BCC. Many old people with aggressive, invasive BCC, which could for example erode a large blood vessel, tend to have other illnesses so that the cause of death is hard to link directly with the BCC. However in a large follow-up series of 2900 BCCs there was a fatality rate of 0.14% directly attributable to the tumour. However, for the 101 patients with recurrent tumour the death rate was 3.9%. Several factors contributed to death in this series (Table 3.2).

Recurrence of basal cell carcinoma

If a BCC appears in the same area as a previously treated tumour it is assumed to represent persistence of the original lesion even when a review of the histology confirms that the original was apparently fully removed. Recurrence

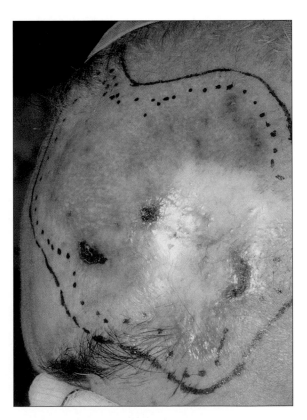

Figure 3.15
Large recurrent basal cell carcinoma with clinical limits of tumour (dotted line) and minimum resection margin (solid line).

Table 3.2
Factors linked to death from basal cell carcinoma.

Primary tumour presenting aged 20–30
Tumour site on central face
Tumour at site of previous radiotherapy

and persistence mean the same in this context. It is sometimes uncertain whether the lesion is a recurrence or a new BCC appearing in the same location. The importance of making this differentiation cannot be overemphasized. Recurrences tend to be larger than the original and have become truly multifocal since several areas of recurrence may occur around and within the scar and deep to the original tumour (Figure 3.15). They are more difficult to treat.

Clinical features

Any change in or around the scar of a previous BCC operation should be taken seriously. Scale or redness, bleeding from the site or more typical BCC appearances are common. Less often the change will be a deep lump, or keloid or cystic lesion but whenever there is doubt a biopsy should be taken.

Time of recurrence

Most recurrent BCCs are recognized within 3 years but some take as long as 20 years to become manifest. Combined statistics from several studies[3] showed that 30% recur in the first year, 20% in the second, 16% in the third, 8% in the fourth and 8% in the fifth. The type of surgical closure also has an influence. In one study most recurrences were seen by the end of the first year if the wound was closed by a full thickness skin graft, by the end of the second year if the wound was closed by a split thickness graft and by the end of the third year for wounds closed by flaps.

Risk factors (see Table 3.3)

While BCC can recur on any part of the body there is a higher incidence on the head and neck than other sites. Clusters occur especially

Table 3.3
Risk factors for recurrence.

Anatomical location – the H zone (Figure 3.16)
Tumour already recurrent
Histological type – infiltrative
Size especially > 2 cm
Experience of initial treating physician
Age – more common in younger patients

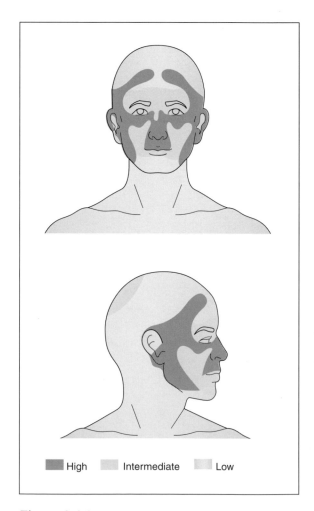

High   Intermediate   Low

Figure 3.16
Relative risk of recurrence at various sites on the head and neck.

on and around the nose, around the eyes, around the ears and on the lateral forehead. Sites of particular concern are around embryonic fusion planes around the ala nasae, the medial and lateral canthi of the eyes and the ears. In these sites there is a greater tendency for tumours to go deep at an earlier stage and to follow embryonic fusion planes and neurovascular bundles. The high-risk areas on the head are shown in Figure 3.16.

The experience of the physician who undertakes the initial treatment is relevant. This is partly explained by the choice of treatment modality, for example whether cryosurgery or excision would be the best option. However experience with a procedure is important. In one study the rate of recurrence for BCC treated by curettage and cautery was 18.8% when carried out by residents but 5.7% when carried out by faculty.

Differential diagnosis

The earliest stage of a BCC may appear as a nondescript tiny papule or an area of nonhealing erosion. The clinical diagnosis is often straightforward but many other lesions come into the differential. Some of these are described here.

Cysts

Superficial epidermoid cysts are whiter than BCC and usually have a punctum (Figure 3.17).

Infected spots

Persistent inflammatory papules are often seen on the head and neck. Generally an antibiotic cream helps the nonmalignant lesions to heal.

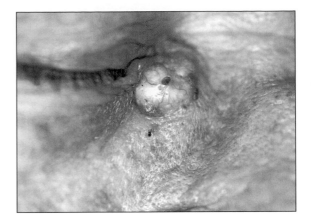

Figure 3.17
Cyst at medial canthus resembling a basal cell carcinoma.

Chondrodermatitis

Prominent areas of the helix or antihelix may develop a nonhealing ulcer secondary to a pressure effect when the ear is pressed against the mastoid bone during sleep. Pain is more common in chondrodermatitis than in BCC and the location on the most prominent area of cartilage is typical. There may be a hypertrophic rim but no telangiectasia.

Sebaceous hyperplasia

These are usually multiple and seen on the forehead, nose and cheeks. The colour is rather yellow especially when the skin is stretched and a tiny central depression may be seen.

Melanocytic naevi

Degrees of pigmentation are common in naevi just as they are in BCC but translucency is rarely a feature. Hairs growing from a lesion are more in keeping with a naevus.

Molluscum

Adults may have a solitary lesion and on the head or neck it may be mistaken for a BCC. With magnification the central keratin core is more obvious.

Warty lesions

Viral warts, small keratoacanthoma, solar keratoses and squamous carcinoma are keratotic. BCCs rarely form true keratin, but often there is a fibrous crust attached and it may be difficult to tell this apart from keratotic lesions. The crust can easily be removed from the surface leaving an eroded base and in this case, it is more likely to be a BCC.

Bowen's disease

It may be impossible to distinguish between BD and BCC. This is particularly so on the lower limbs, but also on the trunk where the superficial type of BCC is often seen. There may be a characteristic whipcord edge to a BCC, but otherwise there is little difference from BD. The diagnostic difficulties have been confirmed in a clinical study.

Tinea

Ringworm may resemble a superficial BCC. The centre may show clearing and tiny pustules can appear at the periphery.

Eczema, psoriasis

Small isolated persistent patches of these inflammatory disorders may be confused with BCC especially the superficial and Bowenoid types. Psoriasis usually has a sharp margin, a silvery scale and small bleeding points which appear on light scratching.

Malignant melanoma

Basal cell carcinoma may be deeply pigmented and shows some features of melanoma. But melanoma may also lack pigment and show some features of a poorly differentiated BCC.

Seborrhoeic keratosis

These great pretenders cause confusion with numerous clinical entities including BCC. The stuck-on appearance, the presence of tiny 'seeds' (keratin pearls) on the surface and sometimes a crumbly nature may help to tell them apart.

Apocrine hydrocystoma

These translucent, blueish, dome-shaped nodules appear around the eye. They tend to be softer than nodular BCC and do not have surface telangiectasia.

Erosions and leg ulcers

One common presentation of BCC is a nonhealing erosion anywhere on the skin. A leg ulcer, which has failed to respond to standard treatment, will occasionally turn out to be a BCC. A readiness to biopsy nonhealing ulcers will prevent falling into this diagnostic trap.

Rarely a BCC will arise in a chronic wound – the Marjolin's ulcer – and again clinical awareness is necessary to reach the diagnosis quickly.

Trichoepithelioma

The solitary form is translucent with surface telangiectasia and is found in the nasolabial folds, cheeks and eyelids. It may be difficult to differentiate clinically and histologically from BCC. Desmoplastic trichoepithelioma is a slow-growing, locally invasive tumour. Most commonly seen on the face, it has a depressed fibrous centre and often a raised, rolled edge providing a difficult differential from infiltrative BCC.

Trichofolliculoma

This may have a central pit but small fluffy hairs will help to define its true nature.

Pilomatricoma

This benign tumour may grow rapidly unlike the usual BCC. They are often dome-shaped with a normal epithelial covering but may have visible flecks of calcification.

Pathology

Basal cell carcinomas occur almost exclusively on hair-bearing skin. They arise from basiloid structures in the epidermis, probably the pluripotential stem cell. They can therefore exhibit differentiating features in several directions and this may account for the wide clinical variability. In particular features of pilosebaceous units and sweat ducts may be seen histologically.

Classification

Many textbooks divide BCC into numerous subtypes but there has been little uniformity. In a recent UK survey 82 histopathologists, from different centres, responded to a questionnaire about classification and excision margins. A quarter had no classification for BCC and the remainder used a wide variety of systems. One system is based on differentiation, another on macroscopic features, the WHO system is very complicated and the others resemble each other quite closely. Without some sort of agreement over classification, it is difficult to compare studies or to plan effective clinical trials. Equally important is the reliance a clinician puts on the pathologist's report to determine the appropriate treatment for each individual. Details from a diagnostic biopsy will help to decide on excision margins and the report on a fully excised specimen will assist in determining prognosis, follow-up policy and counselling of the patient. Below is a simple morphological classification described by Rippey.[4] It combines the best of its predecessors but does not by itself inform on the aggressivity of the tumour. Additional comments may be needed. Two examples of situations not identified are the presence of peripheral palisading and the nature of the most aggressive portion of a mixed pattern BCC.

- nodular, including micronodular,
- infiltrative, including morphoeic,
- superficial, apparently multicentric,
- mixed, including two or more of the above types.

Nodular (approximately 50%)

The common type, which are often clinically nodular, show rounded masses of tumour cells with palisading and often a retraction artefact. Degeneration with cyst formation may be seen. A subgroup with tiny masses, mostly < 0.15 mm, (micronodular) has a higher recurrence rate.

Infiltrative (approximately 15%)

Groups of cells have variable shape and irregular outline and infiltrate between collagen bundles. In the morphoeic subgroup all the cell groups are small and the fibrous stroma is dense, sclerotic and eosinophilic.

Superficial, apparently multifocal (approximately 15%)

Buds of basal cells grow downwards but all remain attached to the epidermis. Despite the normal epidermis seen between the downgrowths, in reality it is a single not a multifocal lesion.

Mixed (approximately 15%)

There may be surprisingly different growth patterns within one tumour, for example, nodular and morphoeic components. This can be misleading if a biopsy is taken from the less biologically aggressive part as it may lead to inadequate treatment.

Additional pathological information

It is of note that a number of features, which may influence the outcome in other malignant tumours, do not appear to affect the prognosis. These include measured depth of invasion, ulceration, degree of inflammation, actinic change, tumour necrosis and nuclear changes such as hyperchromasia, prominence of nucleoli and number of mitoses. Squamous metaplasia with degrees of keratinization may be seen in parts of a BCC. These cells may appear fairly normal, but atypia amounting to carcinoma may also occur: an intermediate cell type has also been recorded. The term basi-squamous carcinoma may be best avoided, recording instead the growth pattern and types of differentiation. If large areas of the tumour show squamous carcinoma, the prognosis may well be more like that of an SCC.

The pathologist may need to distinguish between a BCC showing follicular differentiation and a true hair follicle tumour (trichoepithelioma), and between sebaceous differentiation and a sebaceous epithelioma.

Pigmentation is seen in 2% of BCCs in white-skinned people but in a much higher proportion in black-skinned and Japanese people: they have increased melanocytes and melanophages. It is more common in nodular and superficial tumours and seems to be associated with a higher cure rate as the pigmentation helps to delineate the tumour margins.

Margin of excision should also be recorded, first because it is important to record that the tumour is clear of all margins examined and second to allow the margin and growth pattern to be considered together when deciding on adequacy of treatment and need for follow-up. It may be prudent to follow up a patient with an infiltrative tumour when the margin is as little as 2 mm whereas a small nodular tumour with this margin is highly unlikely to recur.

Diagnostic methods

An experienced clinician will feel confident about the diagnosis in most cases. If there is any doubt a biopsy should be taken. It should provide adequate material for the pathologist to make a diagnosis. Punch biopsy, shave or curette specimens give small samples but may be sufficient in a BCC. Cytotological diagnosis from superficial scrapings have proved a highly accurate and rapid tool for diagnosis.[5] Sometimes when a tumour appears ill defined and Mohs' micrographic surgery (MMS) is not available it can be helpful to take multiple small biopsies around the edge to assess its extent. Finally some clinicians prefer to take a biopsy whenever they are going to embark on a destructive method of treatment which will not provide a specimen, for example, cryotherapy.

Management (see Chapters 7 and 8 for details of techniques and Appendix II for British Association of Dermatologists guidelines)

Prevention

This is discussed fully in Chapter 10. When a BCC has been treated the patient must be informed of the risk of further BCC and offered advice on other sun-related skin disease and an approach to sun protection.

Treatment

Conservative

In very elderly patients or those in poor general health treatment may be unnecessary and unkind. This is especially so for lesions that are unlikely to cause significant problems for the patient in the short term, for example, slow-growing, superficial tumours, especially on the trunk and limbs. Furthermore, some elderly or frail patients with difficult BCCs might prefer less aggressive treatments designed to relieve symptoms of bleeding and discomfort rather than to effect a cure.

Choice of treatment

Choosing the best modality is not always easy. There are many acceptable approaches and the specialist must decide, with a properly informed patient, which is most appropriate for the individual. Each modality has its own risks, limitations, benefits and possible complications. Some patients want to avoid surgery altogether, others want the treatment to be carried out locally and in some there may be important medical conditions which contraindicate a surgical approach. Generally speaking BCCs should always be considered for treatment but the patient has the final decision and must consent. Those who do not want surgery, or those in whom serious medical conditions or drug medication make surgery unsafe, may be considered for a nonsurgical approach. Local availability of specialized services, along with the clinical experience of the specialists involved are other factors likely to influence the selection of therapy.

Rationale of treatment

Basal cell carcinoma is rarely fatal and rarely metastasizes but this does not mean that the cancer can be treated lightly. The problem associated with BCC is its tendency to invade slowly and progressively destroying all local tissues. This applies particularly to tumours of the head and neck. As the cancer grows it develops finger-like extensions which may be invisible to the naked eye but extend several millimetres beyond the clinical margin. These extensions are most commonly found in large lesions, tumours with poorly defined edges (morphoeic) and recurrences. The concept of low- and high-risk tumours is developed further in the next section. The aim of all treatments is to destroy or remove the cancer entirely at the first attempt. If this goal is achieved the BCC will be permanently cured. Otherwise recurrence is likely which is much more difficult to manage.

Low-risk and high-risk basal cell carcinoma

The importance of understanding and recognizing 'low-risk' and 'high-risk' BCC cannot be overemphasized. This knowledge is essential if appropriate treatment is to be given. Basal cell carcinomas vary hugely in their biological and pathological behaviour. Clinical experience allows specialists to look at each patient's skin cancer and decide, according to several criteria, whether simple treatments such as cryosurgery or curettage are likely to be successful (low-risk) or whether more specialized treatments such as wide excision, micrographic surgery or radiotherapy are needed (high-risk).

An example of a low-risk lesion would be a small, primary BCC on the back. It may have clear edges and local spread will be extremely slow: it is unlikely to cause any real harm. A high-risk lesion might be a larger BCC involving the eyelid. It may have poorly defined edges and already be recurrent. This lesion would require careful specialist treatment because of large subclinical extensions and a high risk of further recurrence. Without proper treatment local spread will cause a great deal of harm and eventually lead to loss of the eye. These two situations illustrate that BCCs differ and that no one treatment is best for all lesions.

Factors affecting prognosis

The most important factors affecting prognosis are

- tumour site,
- tumour size,
- definition of clinical margins,
- histological subtype,
- failure of previous treatment,
- immunocompromised host.

Curettage and cautery/electrodesiccation

After curetting the obvious tumour using either a Volkmann spoon or ring curette the edges and base of the wound are cauterized. Variations in the technique such as the number of cycles of treatment, the experience of the operator and careful selection of lesions is crucial to success. Curettage and cautery is best used for low-risk lesions such as small, well-defined, primary lesions usually in non-facial sites and in these cases a 5-year cure rate of up to 97% is possible. It is generally not the best treatment for large tumours, recurrent or morphoeic tumours or tumours in 'high-risk' facial sites such as the periocular area, nose[6] and cheek folds.

Wounds following curettage and cautery heal by secondary intention with cosmetic results which are generally acceptable. The formation of hypertrophic scars can be a problem in certain areas.

Curettage may be performed immediately prior to excisional surgery and helps to define the tumour margins. Prior to cryotherapy it may improve the cure rate.

Cryosurgery

Cryosurgery, usually with liquid nitrogen, is widely used to treat BCC.[7] One or more freeze–thaw cycles may be used and some physicians prefer temperature monitoring. Careful selection of lesions is the key to success; most experts use cryosurgery to treat well-defined lesions away from critical facial sites in order to achieve the best cure rates. Cryosurgery is less effective in treating recurrent BCC. Postoperative wound care can be a problem, as cryosurgery can result in weepy, slow-healing wounds. However, the treatment is usually well tolerated, being performed on outpatients under local anaesthesia, and the cosmetic results can be excellent.

Carbon dioxide laser

This is not widely used in the UK and there is little published follow-up data. It is best for low-risk lesions. When combined with curettage, laser surgery may be useful for large or multiple superficial BCCs, especially on the trunk and limbs.

Surgical excision

The primary objective of excision is to remove the tumour entirely. However, some doctors believe that the total removal of some BCCs may not always be necessary to effect cure. This will be discussed further in the section 'Incompletely excised basal cell carcinomas'. Excision of BCC is normally performed under local anaesthesia, although general anaesthesia may be needed in certain cases. Discussion here is divided into three parts: management of primary (previously untreated), recurrent (previously treated) and incompletely excised lesions.

Primary (previously untreated) BCC: Surgical excision is a highly effective treatment for primary BCC. The cancer and a margin of clinically normal skin around the lesion is included in the excision. The excised tissue can be examined under the microscope and the edges and base of the specimen checked. This is normally on paraffin-embedded sections but occasionally on frozen sections. Wounds can be allowed to heal by secondary intention, closed primarily or repaired with skin flaps or grafts. The overall cosmetic results are usually good. Studies suggest a 95% 5-year cure rate following surgical excision of primary BCC.

What lateral and deep margin of normal skin should be included in the specimen? This question is central to the everyday management of BCC but cannot be answered simply. Many older published papers on BCC recurrence did not detail the margins used. Those that did, usually recommending margins of 2–5 mm, are retrospective. A crucial paper by Wolf and Zitelli described premarking the skin around well-defined tumours with concentric circles at 2 mm increments.[8] Following micrographic excision of the tumours the extent of subclinical tumour invasion was calculated from the presurgical skin markings. A 4 mm margin allowed complete excision of 98% of tumours which were less than 2 cm in diameter. Prognostic factors must be considered for each patient and each tumour before deciding on appropriate margins. The decision about adequate margins should rarely be compromised because the tumour is in a cosmetically sensitive area or because of technical difficulties.

Recurrent (previously treated) BCC: This is essentially the same as for primary lesions, except that it is necessary to remove a larger margin of clinically normal skin from around the BCC: 5–10 mm has been suggested. The 5-year cure rates, probably around 83%, are not as good as for primary lesions.

Incompletely excised BCC: A problem arises if the pathologist reports that the BCC has not been completely removed, especially when the wound is already healing up nicely and there is no obvious sign of BCC on the skin surface. The management of these incompletely excised lesions remains a dilemma. Re-excision of incompletely excised tumours and examination of the margins by horizontal sections shows that up to 55% have residual tumour but this figure cannot be translated into the number which will recur. Some evidence suggests that the total removal of some BCCs may not be necessary to effect cure and that up to two-thirds of incompletely excised BCCs that are not retreated do not recur.[9] Other studies are less optimistic and suggest recurrence rates of up to 50%.[10] There are also different views about the importance of lateral- as opposed to deep-margin involvement.

Patients must be told about the risk of recurrence and the factors involved. Overall it may be reasonable to adopt an expectant policy with BCCs that are incompletely excised on one lateral margin, show nonaggressive histological features, were not previously recurrent tumours and are in noncritical anatomical sites. In contrast, it seems wise to consider retreatment for lesions that are incompletely excised on the deep margin or on two lateral margins, show aggressive histological features, were previously recurrent tumours and are in critical anatomical sites. In this latter situation, re-excision, radiotherapy or MMS are probably the treatments of choice.

Mohs' micrographic surgery

Micrographic surgery allows any residual tumour that is detected to be immediately re-excised, ensuring precise and conservative tumour removal. In more difficult cases the Mohs' micrographic surgeons work with colleagues in ophthalmic and plastic surgery departments allowing patients to benefit from the high cure rates associated with MMS and expert reconstruction of wounds on the face and around the eye. The 5-year cure rate following micrographic excision of primary BCC is around 99% and for recurrent BCC it

is around 94%. Mohs' micrographic surgery is expensive and time consuming, training is arduous and it relies upon specialized technical support. For these reasons it is usually restricted to specialized units in the UK. The treatment is usually reserved for high-risk lesions, especially poorly defined or recurrent lesions involving the eyelids, nose, lips and ears.

Radiation therapy

Radiation therapy is an effective form of treatment for basal cell carcinoma. Success depends upon the skill and experience of the clinical oncologist. Collaboration between dermatologists, plastic surgeons and clinical oncologists in the management of patients with high-risk BCC is a common feature of skin cancer care in British hospitals. As with other forms of treatment, careful patient selection can result in cure rates of around 90% for both primary and recurrent BCC.

Radiation therapy is not ideal for young people as the treatment can produce unsightly changes in the skin some years later with a cosmetic result inferior to that following surgery. It can also be difficult to use radiation therapy to retreat lesions that have already recurred following radiation therapy. Modern therapy has many advantages but may require multiple visits to a specialized unit.

Topical therapy

This mainly involves the use of a cytotoxic drug (5-fluorouracil) in a cream base. This treatment can be used for superficial low-risk BCCs on the trunk and limbs. It is not used to treat more serious lesions. There are insufficient studies to say whether it has a place in the modern management of BCC.

Photodynamic therapy

The role of photodynamic therapy is still the subject of studies and is not widely available in the UK. Long-term follow-up data on large series are not yet available. However, as penetration of the drug appears to be a limiting factor it is likely to be of benefit only for the treatment of superficial lesions in low-risk body sites.

Retinoids

Taken orally they may prevent or delay the development of new BCC. Such therapy has mainly been used in patients with Gorlin's syndrome. Retinoids may also have a lesser effect in producing partial regression of existing lesions. Unfortunately, the relatively high doses needed produce unpleasant side effects, and the BCCs tend to grow back when the treatment is stopped.

Follow-up policy

The overall recurrence rate for BCC is usually quoted at around 5%. When the tumour is apparently fully excised histologically the rate is lower still. This means that following all patients purely to detect recurrence will be an unrewarding experience. Patients with high-risk tumours and those with positive-margin tumours should be followed up.

A different argument is whether to follow patients because of the risk of a second primary. In a 5-year period after excision of a BCC, 36% of patients develop a second primary and 20% develop multiple new BCC.

References

1. Lear JT, Tan BB, Smith AG et al (1997) Risk factors for basal cell carcinoma in the UK: case-control study in 806 patients, *J R Soc Med* **90**:371–4.
2. Ko CB, Walton S, Keczkes K et al (1994) The emerging epidemic of skin cancer, *Br J Dermatol* **130**:269–72.
3. Rowe DE, Carroll RJ, Day CL Jr (1989) Long term recurrence rates in previously untreated basal cell carcinoma; implications for patient follow up, *J Dermatol Surg Oncol* **15**:315–28.
4. Rippey JJ (1998) Why classify basal cell carcinoma? *Histopathology* **32**:393–8.
5. Derrick EK, Smith R, Melcher DH et al (1994) The use of cytology in the diagnosis of basal cell carcinoma, *Br J Dermatol* **130**:561–63.
6. Salasche SJ (1983) Curettage and electrodesiccation in the treatment of midfacial basal cell epithelioma, *J Am Acad Dermatol* **8**:496–503.
7. Holt PJ (1988) Cryotherapy for skin cancer: results over a 5 year period using liquid nitrogen spray cryosurgery, *Br J Dermatol* **119**:231–40.
8. Wolf DJ, Zitelli JA (1987) *Arch Dermatol* **123**:340–4.
9. Dellon AL, DeSilva S, Connolly M et al (1985) Prediction of recurrence in incompletely excised basal cell carcinoma, *Plast Reconstr Surg* **75**:860–71.
10. De Silva SP, Dellon AL (1985) Recurrence rate of positive margin basal cell carcinoma; results of a 5 year prospective study, *J Surg Oncol* **28**:72–4.

Bibliography

Spencer JM, Tannenbaum A, Sloan L et al (1997) Does inflammation contribute to the eradication of basal cell carcinoma following curettage and electrodessication? *Dermatol Surg* **23**:625–31.

Gloster HM, Brodlands DG (1996) The epidemiology of skin cancer, *J Dermatol Surg* **22**: 217–26.

Miller SJ, Maloney ME, eds (1998) *Cutaneous Oncology* (Blackwell Science: Oxford).

Grob JJ, Stern RS, Mackie RM et al, eds (1997) *Epidemiology, Causes and Prevention of Skin Diseases* (Blackwell Science: Oxford).

4 Squamous cell carcinoma

Introduction

Squamous cell carcinoma (SCC) is less common than its basal cell equivalent but it usually has a more aggressive biological behaviour. The incidence is rising along with the other common skin malignancies and to a large extent this is due to increased exposure to ultraviolet radiation. There is a long-running debate about the correct terminology for actinically damaged skin and some people prefer to regard the solar keratosis as an early squamous carcinoma. As there is a continuous spectrum of change from early dysplasia through to invasive disease, breaching the basement membrane, it is not always easy to define an exact cut-off point. However solar keratoses have a very high incidence in the ageing population with some individuals having dozens of lesions. Only a tiny number progress to produce the potentially life-threatening tumours of invasive SCC.

Aetiology and epidemiology

After Sir Percival Pott (1775) had linked SCC to soot as an aetiological agent, Yamagiwa (1915) managed to produce carcinoma experimentally in rabbits using tar. Since then our knowledge of aetiology and understanding of other contributory factors have come on a long way. Today the most important aetiological agent is ultraviolet radiation. Its effects are modified by host, geographical and pigmentary factors.

Incidence

For Caucasians in the USA the incidence of SCC is, per 100 000, 110 in men and 40 in women. There are 1000 deaths each year compared to about 6000 from melanoma.

Host factors

Black-skinned and Asian people have a significantly lower risk of developing SCC. Even within white-skinned groups there are telling differences and southern Italians are at much lower risk than Scandinavians. Fair skin and red hair are independent risk factors as is a tendency to burn rather than tan. Presence of multiple naevi on the back predicts for basal cell carcinoma (BCC) rather than SCC. However the presence of solar elastosis on the neck and telangiectasia on the face were predictors for SCC.

Sunlight exposure

Latitude has a strong relationship to ground levels of incident UVB and equally to the incidence of SCC in the population at those locations. This applies only to immigrant populations rather than the indigenous people. Studies on SCC and occupation have tended to show a positive correlation with those who have a lifetime of occupational exposure suggesting that total lifetime exposure is an important factor in SCC.

Therapeutic radiation and suntanning lamps

UVB is a more powerful carcinogen than UVA but much of the UVB is filtered out by the atmosphere. UVA can augment the effect of UVB. In patients who have had a number of therapeutic UVA courses (usually with psoralens in the treatment of psoriasis, mycosis fungoides etc. in the form of PUVA) the incidence of SCC rises considerably. There is an increased incidence of tumours of the lower extremities. In those who developed SCC after high-dose exposure to PUVA, only 8% of tumours occurred on the head and neck. In a long-term follow-up study more than 25% of patients who were exposed to more than 300 treatments developed one or more SCC. The ratio of squamous to basal tumours is reversed and in men the risk of genital skin cancer rose hugely.

Ionizing radiation

Years ago people with eczema, acne, psoriasis, birthmarks and tinea capitis were at times treated with X-rays. The immediate benefits have been forgotten whereas the rare but serious complication of malignant change has become apparent. Basal cell carcinoma or SCC may occur and although the intervals are very long, the tumour is often aggressive.

Chemical carcinogens

Arsenic has been known to cause malignant change both industrially and when used medicinally for example, Asiatic pills, once used for asthma, and Fowler's solution which was given for psoriasis. The cancer develops years later as a nonhealing ulcer or keratotic nodule usually in nonsun-exposed sites. Distillates of coal and mineral oils may produce SCC.

Immunosuppression

Organ transplant recipients have a high incidence of malignant skin tumours. The normal ratio of BCC to SCC is reversed. The mean interval between transplantation and tumour development is around 7 years: multiple tumours often develop and at an earlier age than expected. The incidence is higher in hot countries, reaching 60% after 20 years in some areas. Many recent reports comment on the biologically aggressive nature of SCC in these patients which is ascribed to the immunosuppressive therapy. The tumours tend to be locally invasive, requiring wide local removal, but there is an increased incidence of metastasis and death. There is no definite link to any particular agent.

Viral infection

Human papilloma virus and herpes simplex have been implicated in the development of SCC. The former may be seen in epidermodysplasia verruciformis, which leads to a selective immunological defect. The role of viruses in SCC is unclear and even when viral DNA is detected in SCC there must be other risk factors acting synergistically.

Scars and chronic inflammation

Burn scars may eventually undergo malignant transformation. This was known long before Marjolin's name became synonymous with malignant change in a variety of scars including leg ulcers, sinuses, osteomyelitis and burns. Since then other chronic inflammatory diseases have also been added to the list. These include tuberculosis of the skin, discoid lupus and both lichen sclerosus and lichen planus especially occurring in genital or perianal skin.

Premalignant lesions

Actinic keratosis is the most common and is discussed in Chapter 2. Porokeratosis, sebaceous naevi and some linear epidermal naevi rarely undergo malignant change.

Genetic syndromes

These are rare syndromes but malignant change, including SCC, can account for a major part of the morbidity. Xeroderma pigmentosa, epidermolysis bullosa, epidermodysplasia verruciformis, poikiloderma congenitale, dyskeratosis congenita and oculocutaneous albinism are the most important.

Natural history

It is worth reading Percival Pott's descripion of squamous carcinoma, starting on the scrotal skin, which is reproduced in Chapter 1. Once malignant, there is an inexorable progression locally with a tendency to metastasize. There is however a wide variation in biological behaviour at different sites and between individuals. Some SCCs begin as solar keratosis on sun-exposed sites and transform slowly into invasive tumours. Some of these hyperkeratotic lesions may remain apparently unchanged for 12–18 months and may not metastasize even when the tumour is many centimetres in diameter. Other SCCs, for example, those on the lip or ear and tumours in immunocompromised individuals may be poorly differentiated and metastasize at an early stage.

Clinical features

Squamous cell carcinoma is a tumour consisting of a progressive growth of contiguous tissue arising from the stratified squamous epidermis (Figure 4.1). It rarely occurs in undamaged skin, being most commonly found on sun-damaged, relatively horizontal cutaneous surfaces, such as the lower lip, top of the ear and scalp of bald men. However because it can develop in areas of chronic inflammation and ulceration SCC may be seen at almost any body site in special circumstances, for example, genital skin in lichen sclerosus and lichen planus.

Differentiation

The proliferative process in an SCC increases the thickness of the skin. This feature may help to differentiate an invasive tumour from a pre-invasive state. The appearance of early lesions will vary according to site and degree of

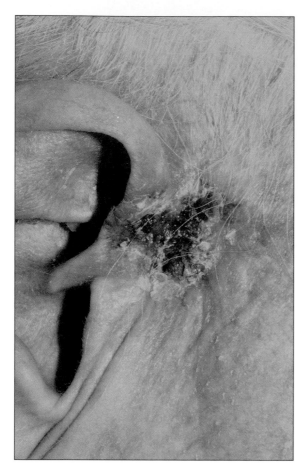

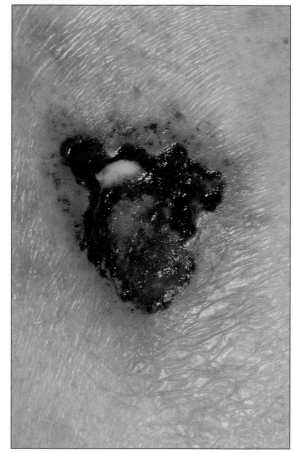

Figure 4.1
Moderately well-differentiated squamous cell carcinoma.

Figure 4.2
Poorly differentiated tumour with characteristic granulation tissue appearance.

differentiation. The typical appearance of an early, well-differentiated carcinoma consists of disorganized keratin, producing a horn in some cases, surmounting a fleshy tumourous base. As the degree of differentiation diminishes so too does the organization of the keratin on the tumour, which may become quite sparse or even absent. In an undifferentiated tumour the stratum corneum may have been replaced by erosion of the surface or frank ulceration. This may appear like granulation tissue (Figure 4.2).

As a tumour enlarges the balance between keratin production and cellular mass shifts towards cellular proliferation (Figure 4.3). Even in a well-differentiated tumour the surface tends to ulcerate and growth takes place predominantly at the margins with an increasing area of granulation tissue occupying the centre (Figure 4.4).

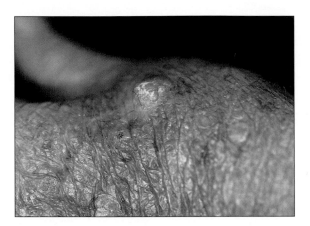

Figure 4.3
Early squamous cell carcinoma with some keratin but increasing cellular proliferation.

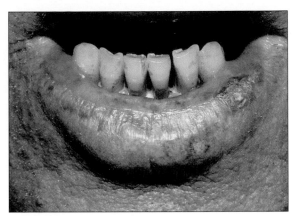

Figure 4.5
Early squamous cell carcinoma of lip.

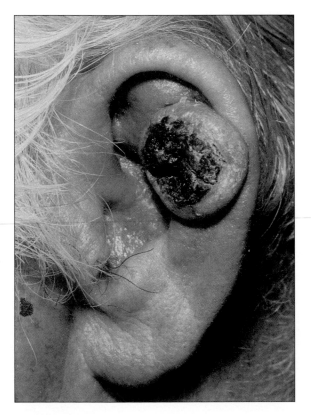

Figure 4.4
Late squamous cell carcinoma of ear with well-developed edge and ulcerated centre.

Mucous membranes

On the lips there are often background changes of actinic cheilitis with an atrophic white mucosa. In this setting early SCC may be hard to diagnose showing minimal induration or ulceration (Figure 4.5). More advanced tumours can be craggy, ulcerated masses (Figure 4.6). In smokers the tumours are more often seen laterally.

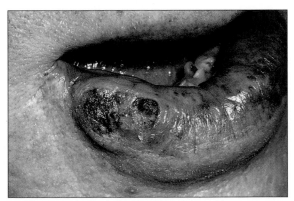

Figure 4.6
Late squamous cell carcinoma of lip.

On the glans penis and vulva, where the epidermis is thin, the earliest sign of SCC is a shallow ulcer possibly with some thickening at the margins

Metastasis

Squamous cell carcinoma may spread in several ways:

- local invasion,
- along tissue planes, between muscles, over perichondrium and periosteum,
- along 'conduits' such as nerve or blood vessels,
- distant metastasis.

Failure to appreciate the tendency of SCC to track will lead to inadequate excision and recurrent tumours. The majority of metastases begin with the local regional lymphatic nodes. Distant metastases are usually by haematogenous spread to the lungs, liver, brain, skin or bone.

Risk factors for metastasis

Most SCCs behave in a relatively benign fashion. Squamous cell carcinoma arising from sun-damaged skin has a low propensity to metastasize, probably around 0.5% compared with 2% for all SCCs of skin. However SCCs arising in certain clinical situations have a much higher rate of spread (Figure 4.7). It is important to be able to recognize the dangerous lesions. Rapid growth is claimed to treble the metastatic rate.

Size and depth

Tumours with a diameter greater than 2 cm have a 5-year cure rate of 72.1% compared

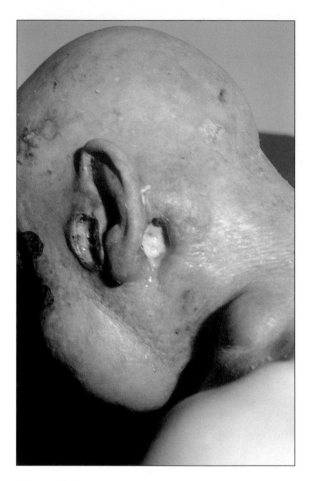

Figure 4.7
Metastatic squamous cell carcinoma after extensive irradiation to head and neck years previously.

with 98.4% for lesions less than 2 cm. The rate of metastasis is probably three times higher. Invasion below Clarke level IV markedly increases the risk of recurrence and metastases, and in one study all tumours resulting in death were more than 10 mm in depth.

Differentiation

Poorly, as opposed to well-differentiated tumours have

- local recurrence rates of 25% compared with 11.8%,
- metastatic rates of 16.4% compared with 6%,
- 5-year cure rate of 61% compared with 94.6%.

Opinions differ as to whether spindle cell SCCs are high-risk, but there is probably a greater incidence of perineural invasion. Adenoid (acantholytic) SCCs are sometimes reported as being aggressive.

Scars and ulcers

Squamous cell carcinoma arising in long-standing scars from radiation, chronic ulceration or infection (for example, osteomyelitis or cutaneous TB) have a risk of metastases from 20 to 40% (Figure 4.8).

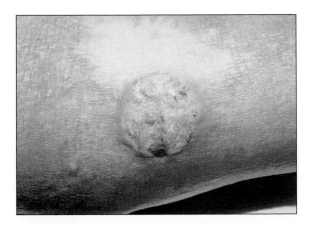

Figure 4.8
Well-differentiated squamous cell carcinoma arising from an old scar.

Site

The lip and the ear are the only sites consistently reported as having a higher risk of metastasis, probably around double that of all sites combined.

Immunosuppression

Immunosuppression increases the risk of tumours in sun exposed skin by up to 21 times, becoming almost universal in the long term. These tumours may have an increased metastatic potential but other factors such as multiple tumours confound the issue.

Perineural invasion

This may occur before symptoms develop, but many reports emphasize a worse prognosis, with local recurrence rates as high as 47% and distant metastases in 34%.

Previous treatment

Local recurrence often carries a poor prognosis. For instance, on the lip, recurrences are associated with 31.5% of metastases and on the ear, 45%.

Factors associated with recurrence

It is important to distinguish between metastasis and recurrence. Many of the factors mentioned above are also relevant in this section but for the surgeon who is attempting to cure an SCC it is necessary to be aware of the biological behaviour of the tumour. The extensions of SCC can be aggressive because they seem to survive without the surrounding stroma necessary for the survival of strands of BCC. They readily invade nerves and move between muscle bundles and other anatomical channels. The appearance of recurrent SCC is highly variable depending on the degree of differentiation of the original tumour, its site and the nature of the surgical procedure and repair.

Size

Subclinical extensions increase with larger tumours. A study with micrographic surgery showed that for tumours less than 2 cm in diameter a 4 mm margin cleared 95% of cases.

Site

The ear is a notorious site for the frequency of recurrence. This is in part because there is a thin dermis so that tumour quickly reaches cartilage and spreads laterally on the perichondrium. Also there is a surgical reluctance to take large margins at this site.

Histology

Poorly differentiated tumours tend to grow more quickly, have larger subclinical extensions and are approximately twice as likely to recur than well-differentiated tumours. Nearly 4% of SCCs demonstrate some tendency for perineural invasion and this is associated with a higher rate of recurrence.

Although verrucous carcinoma is well differentiated it often presents late when it has already burrowed deeply into the tissues and recurrences are common.

Death

Although death from this disease is unusual there are people with aggressive or neglected tumours who die. Retrospective studies tend to show misclassification of certain cases making detailed analysis impossible.

Differential diagnosis

It is important to distinguish SCC from other types of squamous proliferative lesions both benign and malignant. Most SCCs arise on sun-damaged skin and a variety of actinic changes can be expected on the surrounding skin. Signs of sun damage will include the presence of actinic keratoses, lentigines, often quite irregularly shaped, and elastosis with increased skin wrinkling.

Solar keratosis

Some authorities regard solar keratosis as an SCC in situ. When the basement membrane is breached it becomes an invasive carcinoma. It can be impossible to distinguish clinically between some forms of solar keratosis and SCC. Rapid growth and induration at the base may be helpful clues.

Bowen's disease

Both hypertrophic and atrophic ulcerated forms of Bowen's disease (BD) can be confused with SCC. These changes may be seen on the face, hands and legs

Viral warts

Viral warts should not be difficult to diagnose, with their well-organized structure, a collar around the outside and the typical stippled centre. In the elderly however, especially when

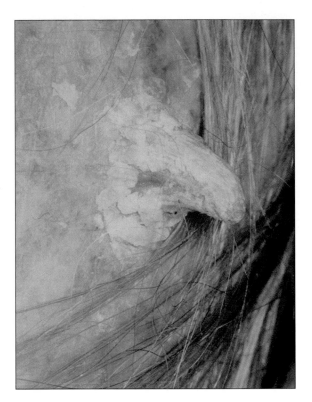

Figure 4.9
Benign cutaneous horn arising from unthickened epidermis.

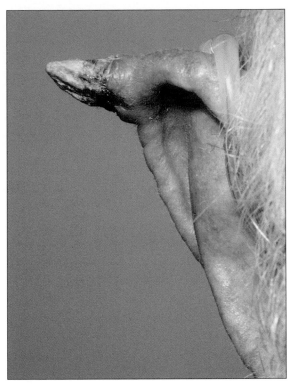

Figure 4.10
Squamous cell carcinoma arising as a cutaneous horn from a thickened and fleshy base.

the warts arise on sun-damaged skin, the difference from a hypertrophic actinic keratosis or early SCC may not be so clear. In the former a smooth, flattened dome with almost normal epidermis covering it helps to differentiate it from both viral warts and SCC.

Cutaneous horn

This may be a manifestation of either a benign or a malignant process. Possible pathologies include viral wart, solar keratosis, BD, seborrhoeic keratosis and SCC. Generally if a horn arises from normal, flat epidermis it is likely to be benign (Figure 4.9). However, if it has a

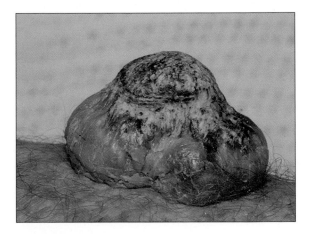

Figure 4.11
Large keratoacanthoma showing collar at base and pouting keratin in centre.

fleshy base, there is a greater chance of malignancy (Figure 4.10). The biological behaviour of the tumour may be helpful in diagnosis: a benign tumour will frequently grow to a limited size but a malignant one tends to continue to enlarge.

Keratoacanthoma

A keratoacanthoma (Figure 4.11) can mimic an SCC but the presence of a neck at the base, the characteristic onion shape and the very rapid growth, developing to several centimetres in diameter in weeks rather than months should make the distinction from SCC clearer.

Basal cell carcinoma

Apart from anaplastic tumours all SCCs are covered with stratified squamous epithelium, the presence of which combined with the absence of radial telangiectasia makes differentiation from nodular and ulcerative BCCs relatively straightforward. Many tumours that resemble Bowen's disease or SCC on the lower leg are histologically confirmed as BCCs.

Leg ulcers

Tumours arising on the lower leg may present particular difficulties in diagnosis, especially when they arise in an area of pre-existing ulceration. The tendency is for such tumours to appear as granulation tissue in an indolent ulcer and indeed it is common for there to be some granulation tissue overlying the SCC. It is therefore important for a very deep diagnostic biopsy to be taken. However there may be a heaped-up edge of irregular keratin especially in a true Marjolin's ulcer.

Pathology

SCC is a tumour of epidermal keratinocytes with nests of prickle cells showing varying degrees of keratinization and horny pearl formation breaking through the basement membrane to invade the dermis. These invading cells may be graded into 'well', 'moderately' and 'poorly' differentiated subtypes, of which the poorly differentiated are the most aggressive and most likely to recur and metastasize. As the tumours dedifferentiate they progress from mature, parakeratotic horny pearls, with individually keratinized cells, towards increasing abnormal mitosis, hyperchromatic nuclei, lessening eosinophilia and tonofibril formation in the cytoplasm. The cells may become more rounded or even spindle shaped. Further classification comprises.

- spindle cell SCC,
- adenoid (acantholytic, pseudoglandular) SCC,
- verrucous carcinoma,
- basi-squamous SCC.

Spindle cell squamous cell carcinoma

These tumours are made up of bundles of spindle cells, which are mostly undifferentiated. They may show evidence of squamous differentiation, but separation from spindle cell melanoma and fibroxanthomas may be difficult, requiring cytokeratin stains, S100 (melanoma positive, SCC negative) and occasionally EM studies.

Adenoid squamous cell carcinoma

This distinctive type has multiple islands or lobules, with nests and columns of gland-like areas caused by acantholysis (dissolution of intercellular bridges) in the centre.

Verrucous carcinoma

Ackerman first described this warty, well-differentiated type in 1948 in the mouth, and the concept has since been extended to the ano-genital region (giant condyloma of Buschke–Lowenstein). These may become huge, cauliflower like and smelly. They are slow growing with marked acanthosis and papillomatosis, with little cytological atypia, usually only invading locally and rarely metastazing unless treated with radiotherapy. Carcinoma (epithelioma) cuniculatum is considered to be the same condition occurring on the plantar surface of the hand or foot.

Basi-squamous squamous cell carcinoma

Basi-squamous carcinomas (also known as metatypical BCCs) have nests of plump squamoid cells, with a tendency to lose the peripheral palisading normally seen in BCCs. Some authors include them with the keratotic type of BCC, with horn cysts. They are relatively rare (probably less that 0.5% of all BCCs) but are much more likely to recur and are the predominating type in the extremely uncommon event of metastasis.

Microstaging and the pathology report

In Chapter 3 the advantages of classifying BCC were discussed. In the pathology report reference to growth pattern and so on is helpful. For SCC it is also useful to report on the degree of differentiation. Breslow depth is also sometimes given. This is routine in malignant melanoma but for several reasons not so common for SCC. Many biopsies simply do not go deep enough to allow this. Also curettage, cryotherapy and radiation do not provide suitable material.

SCC with large tumour islands and which are well circumscribed tend to have small subclinical extensions. Infiltrative tumours with small islands and poor cohesion are more difficult to define and tend to recur more often. Perineural and perivascular invasion indicate a more aggressive tumour which will be more difficult to eradicate.

Diagnostic methods

Very well-defined tumours which clinically may be a solar keratosis variant rather than an SCC may be diagnosed and treated by curettage or deep shave excision. If the histology suggests a more aggressive SCC then wider excision can be performed.

The approach for larger and less well-differentiated tumours is not so clear. Many specialists make a clinical diagnosis and plan excisional surgery with margins determined by size, site and age. However a diagnostic biopsy is another good approach. It should be deep into the subcutis to allow the pathologist to report on the depth.

Management (see British Association of Dermatologists guidelines – Appendix III)

Prevention

This is covered more fully in Chapter 9. The patient must be made aware of the need to protect the skin from excess ultraviolet indefinitely. Also the risk of further skin malignancy must be explained. In one study[1] 30% of SCC patients developed additional SCCs and 52% developed subsequent nonmelanoma skin cancer within 5 years of therapy for their first SCC.

Conservative

In the discussion of BCC treatment a case was made for conservative management in certain situations. This applied particularly to frail elderly people with biologically nonaggressive tumours. This is less often possible with SCC because a greater proportion of the tumours are aggressive with the potential to metastasize. However there are some lesions, such as hyperkeratotic horns on the back of the hand or on the scalp, the histology of which would probably be SCC, which can be left alone if the patient is frail or in a home.

Principles of treatment

The intention must always be to cure the patient of the primary tumour and to prevent metastasis. The factors that can affect the rate of recurrence and the chance of metastasis have been discussed earlier in the chapter and must be taken into account when planning the treatment. Part of the assessment may be to take a pretreatment biopsy to ensure that it is indeed an SCC but also to get further information about the degree of differentiation, the presence of vascular invasion and so on.

As with other skin cancers no one form of treatment has been shown to be effective in all cases and treatment should be tailored to the individual as much as possible. With SCC it has been shown that all the risk factors for recurrence and metastasis, except host immunosuppression, are linked to subclinical extension of the primary tumour. The inescapable conclusion is that poor prognosis is linked to inadequate destruction of the primary tumour.

Comparing the success of one modality to another must allow for the differences in the tumours included in the study. If one investigator is treating SCCs larger than 2 cm and in sites where wide clearance is technically difficult it is unhelpful to compare the recurrence rate with a group of low-risk, smaller tumours. Some of the dermatological literature relates to large studies where the SCC are well differentiated, diagnosed at an early stage, in patients undergoing regular review and treated successfully with modalities such as cryotherapy or curettage and cautery. The recurrence rate cannot be compared usefully with a study of large, poorly differentiated tumours, requiring wide excision and postoperative radiotherapy, where cure may be hard to achieve.

Multidisciplinary oncology team

In any hospital there will be specialists who are able to deal with SCC at different sites. It is important that none of these experts work in isolation. The concept of a multidisciplinary team has gained a consensus approval over the last few years. It allows discussion of all cases in an environment which encourages pathological review prior to reasoned treatment planning. A clinical oncologist, dermatologist, pathologist and appropriate surgeon should be on the team.

Curettage and cautery (for details of technique see Chapter 7)

The choice of lesion is paramount with this technique. It is generally agreed that small, well-differentiated, superficially invasive, nonrecurrent SCC are best suited for this method. The literature is full of studies showing excellent cure rates, sometimes up to 100% in the right hands. Ideal lesions would be the hyperkeratotic nodules that may appear on the dorsum of the hand or scalp. It is often recommended that a 2–5 mm margin is included to destroy subclinical tumour spread. If a pretreatment biopsy is taken it should be a shave not a punch so that the curette does not delve into the hole. Although curettage is not generally recommended for larger or poorly differentiated SCC, there is little high quality published evidence either to encourage or discourage its use. In a 1998 paper[2] SCC of the external ear measuring up to 23 mm were treated by curettage followed by a double freeze–store cycle with liquid nitrogen. There were no recurrences and all patients were followed for 2–5 years. The ear is often regarded as a high-risk area so presumably the curette must have helped to debulk and delineate the tumour to allow maximum benefit from the cryosurgery. Certainly the principle of debulking before cryosurgery is well accepted.

Cryosurgery

The combination of cryosurgery and curettage is a logical approach and is mentioned in the previous section. It is sensible to debulk a hyperkeratotic SCC prior to cryosurgery because keratin is a good insulator. Its use in poorly differentiated, nonkeratinizing SCC is less common. Despite numerous small studies to support the use of cryosurgery and the huge amount of clinical experience in some hands, there are no long-term prospective studies to date. Cryosurgery may have a special place in the very elderly who may be confined to a residential home.

Laser

Lasers may be used as excisional instruments with the advantage of sealing small blood vessels and lymphatics. Surgery may be easier in vascular areas and theoretically may decrease the dissemination of tumour cells. Disadvantages are increased cost, safety hazards and unwieldy delivery systems. Their place is limited in the treatment of SCC.

Photodynamic therapy

There are a few small studies using systemic porphyrin photodynamic therapy for SCC but currently it is not an accepted method of treatment.

Retinoids

Etretinate and Isotretinoin have been used but the latter is often preferred for its shorter half-life. The main indication is the prevention of new tumours in immunosuppressed patients, is often following organ transplantation. It has to be used long term but side-effects such as dryness of the lips may be a problem. Higher doses of Isotretinoin, for example, 1 mg/kg may be better especially if the indication is for advanced recurrent disease.

Excision

Excisional surgery is suitable for small and large lesions alike and at any site. It is reassuring because the pathologist is able to examine the entire surgical specimen and comment on the adequacy of tumour removal. This is not a foolproof system because it gives no information about metastases or lymphatic spread.

Nor does routine histopathology give as much information as micrographic surgical sections. Following excision healing is generally quick and cosmetic results are good but large defects may require difficult reconstruction.

Some surgeons prefer to leave the surgical wound open until the pathologist's report is back. The excised specimen can be marked with a suture at one end to help with orientation: this may be useful if further tissue needs to be removed because the tumour has been incompletely excised. Though not as scientific as micrographic surgery, this is a sensible approach especially for ill-defined tumours.

The excision margin will vary depending on the size, site, histological features and whether it is a primary or recurrent tumour. There are no good prospective studies to help with decision making. The wealth of clinical experience and retrospective studies which have been published give indicators but often the studies omit details of margins, tumour size or site or degree of differentiation. Margins between 2 and 10 mm are generally agreed upon. In a helpful paper Brodland and Zitelli[3] used micrographic surgery to demonstrate what minimum margins were required for histological clearance. For well-differentiated tumours smaller than 2 cm, not in high-risk sites and not involving fat, a 4 mm margin was adequate. For poorly differentiated tumours the margin was 6 mm if they were more than 2 cm in diameter in low-risk sites or more than 1 cm in high-risk sites.

There is still debate about how to close large defects after SCC removal. Historically skin grafts have been advocated because flaps may hide recurrent tumour for a long time. The surgeon will be more confident using a flap if the pathologist's report is back before closure – either by delaying closure for routine histology or using micrographic surgery.

Mohs' micrographic surgery

The same principles apply to SCC and BCC (see Chapter 3). There is maximum preservation of normal tissue and maximum chance of eradicating all the tumour. There are good studies to show high cure rates of up to 97% and even 99.5% of SCC less than 1 cm in diameter. As with other techniques the poor prognostic variables adversely affect a cure rates. For most clinicians the argument is not whether Mohs' micrographic surgery (MMS) should be available as an option but for which patients it is most suitable. There are some who advocate its use for all high-risk lesions linked to size, site and histology. Others would only resort to MMS for very large or recurrent lesions.

Radiation therapy

The balance between preservation of healthy tissues and destruction of tumour is important not only in terms of effectiveness and healing time but also the cosmetic result. Radiation is useful either as the sole treatment or combined with surgery. Electron-beam therapy has increasingly found favour for treatment of skin cancer compared to superficial X-rays, because it provides a more uniform dose from the surface to the desired depth and more rapid fall-off which protects underlying tissues.

The cure rates are much better for smaller tumours. Several studies, using a variety of fraction size, total dose and X-ray energy have shown that for tumours of 2 cm or less, the 5-year cure rate is about 98%, for tumours 2–5 cm around 90% and for tumours over 5 cm as low as 60%. Radiation may also be offered after incomplete surgical excision or where the clinical situation suggests that lymph nodes may be involved. In this context radiation has been shown to reduce the rate of local recurrence.

Special sites

Although SCCs on the lip may keratinize, their biological behaviour is somewhere between that of SCC on the skin and those on mucous membranes (which are more aggressive): they have a rate of metastasis almost twice as much as other skin sites. In advanced tumours this is nearly 90%. The ear is another area with a reputation for early metastasis. Lesions on the external auditory meatus and concha are much more likely to invade bone at an early stage than those of the helical rim.

Follow-up policies

Seventy-five per cent of SCCs which recur do so within 2 years and 95% of recurrences are within 5 years. For this reason most clinicians advocate some form of follow-up for at least 4 years. This should probably be every 3 months for the first year and 6 months thereafter. Close examination of the surgical site and draining lymph node areas is recommended.

References

1. Frankel D, Hanusa B, Zitelli J (1992) New primary non melanoma skin cancers in patients with a history of squamous cell carcinoma of the skin, *J Am Acad Dermatol* **26**:720–6.
2. Nordin P (1998) Curettage–cryosurgery for non melanoma skin cancer of the external ear; excellent 5 year results, *Br J Dermatol* **140**:291–3.
3. Brodland DG, Zitelli JA (1992) Surgical margins for excision of primary cutaneous squamous cell carcinoma, *J Am Acad Dermatol* **27**:241–8.

Bibliography

Johnson TM, Rowe DE, Nelson BR, Swanson NA (1992) Squamous cell carcinoma of the skin (excluding lip and oral mucosa), *J Acad Dermatol* **26**:467–84.

Dinehart SM, Pollack SV (1989) Metastasis from squamous cell carcinoma of the skin and lip, *J Acad Dermatol* **21**:241–8.

Petter G, Haustein U-F (2000) Histologic subtyping and malignancy assessment of cutaneous squamous cell carcinoma, *Dermatol Surg* **26**:521–30.

5 Primary malignant melanoma

Definition

Malignant melanoma (MM) is a tumour arising chiefly from melanocytes of the basal layer of the epidermis and less often from extracutaneous sites such as the uveal tract and meningeal membranes.

Introduction

Malignant melanoma – the 'malignant mole' – plays lead role in the demonology of those who specialize in treating diseases of the skin. It creates fear not only in patients afflicted with this cancer but also in clinicians involved with their care. There are many reasons for this, some of which are all too real, while others are part of the mythology that has built up around this malignancy.

The incidence and to a lesser degree the mortality of cutaneous MM appeared to increase at an alarming rate during the latter half of the twentieth century, almost reaching epidemic proportions in Queensland, Australia in the early 1980s. Early tumours are usually curable by simple surgical excision, however once they have spread this cancer is very difficult to treat. Malignant melanoma accounts for approximately 10% of all skin cancers, however it is the cause of 80% of the deaths due to skin cancer. There are other features of MM that cause it to be so feared. It is a disease that predominately affects white-skinned people of north European descent, it can arise at an early age and affects people in the higher socio-economic groups. These facts together with its association with recreational sun exposure have led MM to be perceived as a disease that strikes down young white Caucasian adults who are otherwise in the prime of their lives, and is the result of their enjoyment of their hard-earned leisure time. This group forms a particularly vociferous population with the resources to publicize and research the disease.

The challenge of managing MM has increased to the extent that in Australia, the country with the highest incidence of MM, it has become the fourth most common cancer in both men and women. In North America it is the tenth most common and in the UK it is the eighteenth most common cancer. The reduction in mortality from MM has become a prime goal for public health campaigns. To achieve this it is necessary to separate reality from myth of MM so that the true risk factors for the development of MM can be identified and thus give a clear and unambiguous message about prevention. Better management of both early and advanced disease will only come from a better understanding of the biology of the tumour.

Aetiology and epidemiology

Rising incidence

The incidence of melanoma varies greatly around the world and between different racial groups. There is compelling evidence that there has been a true increase in incidence and to a lesser degree mortality from MM in the developed world. This evidence is gained from numerous cancer registries which have recorded information on both the incidence and mortality of MM over many years. This has revealed an increase in incidence of between 3 and 7% per year between the early 1960s and the late 1980s in populations of European descent. This rise in incidence reached dramatic proportions during the 1980s with a doubling of incidence in a 2–3-year period in certain populations notably in Scotland,[1] Australia and New Zealand. This change has not been seen (with the possible exception of Japan) in non-European populations. Encouragingly recent evidence indicates that this rise in incidence may have reached a plateau in the USA, Scotland and Australia and may actually be falling in females.

The rapid rise in incidence in the 1980s coincided with heightened interest of both health care professionals and patients in the disease and the excision of many more pigmented lesions. The majority of the increases in reported MMs were of thin ones and it has been postulated that many of these early thin MMs are actually nonprogressor lesions and as such have artificially boosted incidence rates. The implication is that histological reporting of certain worrying features has become removed from the biological reality of the tumour.

Unfortunately this is not a theory that can be confirmed or refuted; with our present knowledge it would not be ethical to simply observe such lesions to see what happens to them. Despite this there is little doubt that the long-term trend in incidence rates has been upward and it is mirrored by an increase in mortality from MM.

Skin colour and ethnicity

A critical review of the data on incidence rates reveals further clues to the causes of MM. The most striking data show that it is predominately a disease of white Caucasians, the lowest incidence of 0.5 per 100 000 person-years occurs in Asia and in the African American population in the USA. This compares to the highest incidence of approximately 27 per 100 000 person-years in Australia. This relationship is even more striking when differences in sunburn potential and ability to tan are taken into account. Among Europeans living in Europe there are wide differences in incidence of MM. The lowest incidence is seen in people living in southern Italy and Spain, and the highest rates are found in Scandinavia and in those people of Celtic origin in the UK.

Thus there appears to be an inverse relationship between skin pigmentation and risk of MM. This relationship also holds for hair colour and to a lesser extent eye colour, with red hair and blue eyes conferring the greatest risk for developing MM. The receptor for the melanocyte-stimulating hormone can exist in different 'polymorphic' forms; certain polymorphisms are more frequently found in 'sun-sensitive' individuals and may lead to the development of genetic markers of these at-risk individuals.

Different populations may produce different types of melanin in response to ultraviolet radiation; black-skinned individuals produce eumelanin which is far more protective than the phaeomelanin produced by the classic Celtic phenotype. Indeed there is evidence that phaeomelanin may actually enhance the mutagenic potential of ultraviolet radiation.

Geographical and ultraviolet exposure

Another striking fact is the increase in incidence with increasing proximity to the equator: this is especially apparent in Australia and the USA where relatively homogeneous white populations are spread over broad bands of latitude. This supports the causative role of ultraviolet radiation in the pathogenesis of MM. However this relationship is not so straightforward as it is, for example, with squamous cell carcinoma (SCC).

The confounding data of a higher incidence of MM in Scandinavia as opposed to southern Europe can be explained by the difference in skin type between these populations. Careful case-control studies performed in Australia, Canada and Denmark have also shown that excess sun exposure is related to an increased risk of developing MM. However when these data are looked at more closely the picture becomes less clear. Unlike SCC, MM is not a disease related to higher cumulative exposure to ultraviolet radiation. Indeed MM is more commonly seen in people who have indoor occupations. Thus the concept of intensity of exposure became important. Studies that have looked at intermittent, high-intensity exposure, such as that experienced by office workers during their two weeks' holiday to the sun, and also at episodes of sunburn, have shown a positive association with the development of MM. Unfortunately most of the studies looking at levels of sun exposure and episodes of sunburn are at risk of recall bias and this questions the validity of the data.

There is interesting variation in the site of origin of MM between the sexes in white Caucasians, with most MMs developing on the trunk in men and the lower legs in women. Initially this led to the hypothesis of a 'solar circulating factor' induced by ultraviolet radiation on exposed sites which promoted MM development at distant sites. However this has now been largely discounted and this variation in site of origin is now thought to relate more to intermittent high-intensity exposure at these sites.

Migration studies offer an interesting refinement on the risks of sun exposure. They show that white Caucasians who are born in areas of low incidence of MM and move to sunnier climates with a higher incidence of MM, tend to have a lower incidence of MM than the native residents with similar skin type. This difference is not seen if the migration occurs during the early years of life. Before the age of 10 children appear to adopt the higher risk of developing MM if they move into areas with higher incidence rates.

Family history

The majority of MMs occur in a sporadic pattern, however between 2 and 10% of patients presenting with MM give a positive family history of one or more first degree relatives with MM. The study of these relatives with MM provides further insight into the possible causes of MM. In part this phenomenon may be due to the inheritance of specific MM susceptibility genes. A germline mutation in a gene CDKN2A, which encodes for the production of a protein that inhibits cell division, has been identified on chromosome 9 in certain of these relatives with MM. In other families with a very strong history of MM this gene has not been isolated and the search for other genes implicated in the development of MM continues.

Another explanation for the familial clustering of MM is the grouping of other known risk factors such as skin type, number of naevi and sun exposure. Using segregation analysis it has been shown that Mendelian inheritance of one major susceptibility gene cannot explain the familial clustering of MM in a large population-based study in Australia. Indeed it would appear that specific gene mutations account for only a fraction of the familial MMs.

Congenital naevi

About 1% of newborns have congenital naevi. They tend to be larger in size than acquired naevi, with deeper extension of melanocytes into the dermis and surrounding appendages. Clinically these have been subdivided into estimated adult sizes of small (< 2 cm), intermediate and large/giant (> 20 cm).

An increased risk of MM has been attributed to small congenital naevi and, although this risk has not been accurately defined, it is believed to be small.[2] A complicating factor in the assessment of the risk of congenital naevi is the fact that some of the acquired naevi appearing during infancy and early childhood are indistinguishable, clinically and histologically, from truly congenital naevi.

Giant naevi are uncommon, occurring in less than 1 in 20 000 newborns. They are typically irregularly pigmented with a multinodular texture and course hairs. Multiple smaller satellite naevi may be present at birth and can develop in infancy. Neural melanosis with melanocytic proliferation within the leptomeninges and brain parenchyma may be present when giant lesions overlie the head and spine. The lifetime risk of MM or other neural crest malignancies in giant naevi is estimated at 5–15%.[3] Satellite naevi have not been associated with malignant change and giant naevi centred on limbs may carry a lower risk.

Acquired melanocytic naevi

Often a positive history of a preceding mole can be gained when patients present with MM. In addition when histological sections of MM are studied an associated naevus is often seen. Taken together these data give estimates that between 30 and 50% of all MMs arise in pre-existing naevi.

In foetal life melanocyte migrates from the neural crest to the basal layer of the epidermis junction. The three main types of acquired melanocytic naevi, junctional, compound and intradermal naevi, are believed to derive from these basal layer melanocytes and represent a maturation process. These melanocytes become naevus cells and proliferate in continuity with the dermoepidermal junction to produce the small, macular, brown junctional naevus. With time groups of melanocytes detach from the dermoepidermal juction and lie in the dermis whilst retaining a junctional component. This is then called a compound naevus which is usually light tan to brown and is a raised, palpable lesion. Again with time the junctional component is lost and there are melanocytes in the dermis only. These are called intradermal naevi and are small, fleshy, palpable lesions with little or no pigment. Thus the majority of naevi in children are junctional naevi, in young adults compound naevi and in older adults intradermal naevi. The number of melanocytic naevi gradually increases from 6 months of age to the third decade of life, after which there is a gradual decline so that 70–80-year-old patients have few or none.[4] The anatomic distribution of and the rate of change in the number of melanocytic naevi is in part a function of ultraviolet radiation. Mole counts in identical twins are highly concordant suggesting a genetic influence. Immunosuppressed children and those who have undergone treatment for cancer also acquire increased numbers of naevi.

There are now convincing data that increased numbers of acquired melanocytic naevi confer an increased risk of MM; indeed several studies show a linear relationship between number of naevi and MM risk. When compared with other risk factors, the total number of all melanocytic naevi provides the most significant risk factor for the development of MM.

When studying the role of naevi in the development of MM there exists an ambiguity in the relationship between the number of moles and skin type. The fact that more naevi are seen on lighter skin types has led to the supposition that they are induced by excess sun exposure in individuals with increased sun sensitivity. Conversely it may indicate that the genes controlling phenotypic characteristics are closely allied to those controlling the number of naevi. The relationship between number of naevi and risk of MM still holds even if these other phenotypic characteristics are controlled for. It appears that sun exposure, particularly in the first 20–30 years of life promotes the development of naevi and that sun-sensitive skin types have more of these acquired naevi; however, whether this is due to an individual's inherent ability (or lack of) to block ultraviolet radiation or to their degree of activation of the melanocyte system remains unanswered.

Atypical naevi and the atypical naevus syndrome

Most acquired naevi are small (less than 5 mm in diameter), evenly pigmented and with a regular border. Occasionally moles are encountered that are strikingly different; these 'atypical' naevi are larger, often with bizarre irregular outlines. Histologically they have the appearance of compound naevi but individual melanocytes and even nests of melanocytes may exhibit cytological atypia. It has been postulated that these lesions are precursor lesions for MM; however the evidence supporting this is weak. Whereas common melanocytic naevi appear primarily in the first few decades of life, it is believed that atypical moles develop throughout life.[5]

For many years an association between a familial occurrence of MM and an atypical naevus phenotype has been noted. Patients with this phenotype not only have large numbers of naevi but in addition they have significant numbers (more than two) of clinically atypical naevi and naevi in unusual places such as the buttocks, anterior scalp and iris of the eye. With the absence of a reliable genotypic marker of increased risk of developing MM this atypical naevus phenotype does indicate an increased risk of developing MM although as a marker it has low sensitivity.

Lentigo maligna

This is discussed more fully in Chapter 2. These flat, irregularly pigmented lesions usually develop on the head and neck of elderly people. They have approximately a 10% risk of eventually producing a vertical growth phase and when that happens the disease progresses as an MM elsewhere.

Occupation

Most data on occupational risk suffer from lack of control for phenotype, mole counts and sun-exposure history. Hazardous chemicals in the work place could not account for many cases of MM, indeed in the USA men with 'white collar' jobs are more at risk of developing MM. The difference in risk between different occupations has more to do with different lifestyles rather than work place factors.

Exposure to artificial sources of ultraviolet radiation such as fluorescent lighting and tanning lamps has been blamed as a cause of MM but only weak associations have been found.[6] Such studies are confounded by the fact that many of those who use sunbeds also spend excessive time trying to achieve a tan in natural sunshine.

Sunscreens

Sunscreens have been promoted as protective agents to reduce the incidence of MM. Unfortunately this is not supported by epidemiological data. Indeed there is some information that sunscreen use may actually increase the risk of MM. This finding may point to a direct causal role of sunscreen chemicals in the development of MM, although it appears far more likely that their use has a permissive role in allowing more prolonged exposure to the sun in patients at risk. It may also indicate that longer wavelengths of ultraviolet radiation (UVA) play a more important role in the development of MM as these wavelengths are more difficult to block.

Water pollution

Recently attention has been paid to the role of water pollution in the development of MM. This theory would help to explain the relationship between intermittent sun exposure and MM because sun exposure and water sports are highly correlated. There is evidence that people who learn to swim before the age of nine and who indulge in regular swimming activities both in swimming pools and open water have an increased risk of developing MM. This may be due to halogenated compounds found in water as these products are known to cause pigment–cell neoplasms, chromatophoromas, in fish.

Oral contraceptive pill

Oestrogen taken for contraception or for postmenopausal hormone replacement is known to cause increased skin pigmentation, and oestrogen receptors (or the capacity to bind oestrogens) have been found on MM cells. These facts together with the observation that MM in women increases from puberty but starts to level off after the menopause, led researchers to investigate the role of the oral contraceptive in the aetiology of MM. Although the most recent data have failed to show an association between the use of the oral contraceptive pill (OCP) and MM, further research is needed to clarify the role of long-term OCPs, hormone replacement and reproductive events in MM development.

Iatrogenic causes

The incidence of MM is higher in patients who are on high-dose immunosuppression following organ transplant surgery, and patients who have had an MM excised before transplantation are more likely to develop metastases. PUVA photochemotherapy has been shown to increase the risk of developing nonmelanoma skin cancer, however an increased risk of developing MM has not been proven.

Table 5.1
Risk factors for melanoma.

Large numbers of benign naevi
Freckles
Clinically atypical naevi
Severe sunburn
Early years in a tropical climate
Family history of MM

Relative risk

Four independent risk factors for the development of MM have been identified by the Scottish Melanoma Group. The most important independent risk factor in the northern European Caucasian population is the total number of benign naevi (Table 5.1). The additional three independent risk factors are the presence of lentigines (freckles), the presence of three or more clinically atypical melanocytic naevi and a history of three or more episodes of severe sunburn. In this case-control study the traditional risk factors of fair or red hair, blue eyes and fair skin were surrogates for the tendency to develop naevi and freckles and to burn in the sun.

To put some of these risks into perspective, every red-haired individual has a relative risk of developing an MM of 3. The estimated relative risk of developing an MM in an individual with atypical mole syndrome (AMS) and no family history is 7 whereas at the other end of the spectrum, an individual with AMS and a family history of two MMs has a relative risk of around 500.[7]

Natural history

It is only possible to diagnose MM with certainty when it has been excised or if it has shown its malignant nature by local spread or metastasis. There is therefore little opportunity to observe the natural history of early disease. However there are still a few patients who have very large superficial MM, for example, more than 5 cm in diameter, present for many years and in whom no local spread has occurred. There may be others with small lesions which have not progressed over the years. Overall however it is assumed that untreated MM will inevitably go on to metastasis and death. Despite treatment 25% of people will eventually die of their disease.

Metastasis can occur at an early stage but lie dormant for years before manifesting itself. The immune system must have suppressed growth at the distant site in the intervening years. The presentations of metastatic disease are protean. The classic description of advanced disease is found in Chapter 1.

Clinical features

(including differential diagnosis)

The clinical evaluation of patients with suspected MM includes a careful history of the lesion concerned and an examination of all the patients' pigmented lesions. The main diagnostic feature of MM is the history of change in a pigmented lesion, usually over a period of 2–6 months. A very short history of change suggests trauma, haemorrhage into the skin (Figure 5.1) or inflammation. Bleeding, oozing and crusting are rare in early MM but occur as the tumour becomes thicker. Pain is not a feature of primary MM. Itch on its own is not a significant symptom but in association with other suspicious features it may be helpful. The key to the clinical diagnosis of a

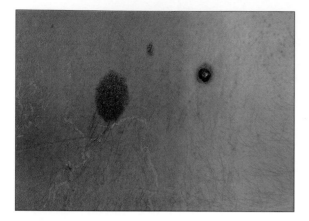

Figure 5.1
Right-hand lesion changed very quickly and histology showed bleeding into a haemangioma.

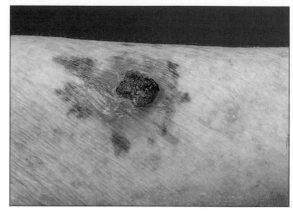

Figure 5.2
Irregularity of colour is an important feature.

pigmented MM is irregularity of the lesion. Irregularity of colour is important and the presence of a variety of colours in one lesion is highly suspicious (Figure 5.2). Black, brown, red, grey and white all occur: partial regression leads to some loss of pigment, inflammation causes redness and dermal invasion gives blue/black hues.

Irregularity of the outline is the second most important feature and MM may demonstrate indentations or 'notches' as well as outgrowths around the perimeter of the lesion (Figure 5.3). Two systems have been devised to aid in clinical diagnosis of MM: the Glasgow Seven Point Check List and the American ABCDE System.

In the Glasgow system there are three major and four minor features:

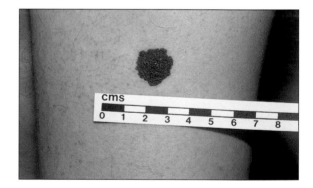

Figure 5.3
Notched irregular border is one feature of malignant melanoma.

Major	(1)	Change in size
	(2)	Irregularity of pigmentation
	(3)	Irregularity of outline

Minor	(4)	Diameter greater than 6 mm
	(5)	Inflammation
	(6)	Oozing or bleeding
	(7)	Itch or altered sensation

It is suggested that any lesion with one major feature in an adult be considered for excision biopsy. The presence of the minor features will add to the suspicion that MM is occurring. This system is mainly used in the UK. The American ABCDE system is as follows:

Asymmetry — Opposite segments of the lesion are appreciably different.

Border — Border is irregular resembling a coastline with bays and promontories. Usually well defined in MM unlike dysplastic naevus where the border is often ill defined, fading into normal skin.

Colour — Colour variation. A narrow red halo may be seen around an MM. Amelanotic MM will have little or no distinguishing colour.

Diameter — Superficial spreading MM is usually greater than 6 mm in diameter.

E — E was originally for 'elevation' but missed some early MM. E is now for 'examination' of other lesions. The MM is usually different from the patient's other moles. Also a second primary MM may be detected.

The presence of hair does not exclude a diagnosis of MM. However in thicker MMs, hair will disappear as the invading tumour destroys the follicles. Thick MMs feel firm to the touch, not soft or compressible like haemangiomas. Some MMs have a surrounding halo of depigmentation. This is not diagnostic of MM as it occurs frequently in benign naevi (halo or Sutton's naevus). In MM the depigmentation, like the lesion itself, tends to be highly irregular compared to the regular halo around a benign naevus.

The appreciation of the clinical features of pigmented lesions of the skin can be enhanced by the use of surface microscopy (dermatoscopy, dermoscopy, epiluminescence). This technique uses a light magnification system ($\times$ 10) with immersion oil at the skin microscope lens interface. The use of oil prevents the scattering of light by the skin scales of the stratum corneum and allows the epidermis to become translucent. Thus a detailed examination of the pigmented and vascular structures of the epidermis and upper dermis can be made, revealing many features not visible to the naked eye. It is possible to identify patterns of melanin distribution and the vascular nature of haemangioma is blatantly demonstrated. With training and experience, useful clues can be gleaned from dermatoscopy, to add to the clinical impression. However at present dermatoscopy is only an aid to diagnosis and if there is clinical suspicion, biopsy and histological examination of the pigmented lesion remains the key to the definitive diagnosis.

The original division of MM into three clinicopathological subgroups (superficial spreading malignant melanoma (SSMM), nodular (NM) and lentigo maligna melanoma (LMM)) by Clark et al in 1969 and the addition of a fourth subgroup, acral lentiginous melanoma by Reed et al in 1975 was initially thought to correspond to different types of MM. Initially the different subgroups were thought to have distinct behaviour and prognosis. However it is now recognized that these clinicopathological variants are not independent prognosticators. The outcome is strictly dependent on the Breslow thickness of the tumour whatever the subgroup. However the clinical differences in the four main subgroups warrant their preservation as the distinct clinical features of each subgroup give rise to a different range of lesions to be considered in the differential diagnosis.

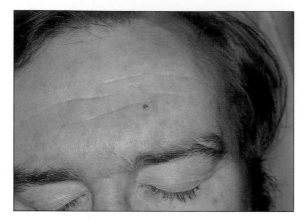

Figure 5.4
An early superficial spreading melanoma.

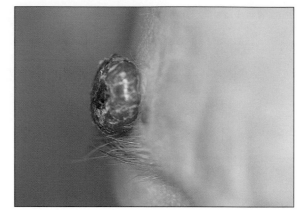

Figure 5.5
Thick nodular malignant melanoma.

Superficial spreading malignant melanoma

This is the most common type of MM seen in the white-skinned population, comprising 70% of cases and presenting most frequently in the fourth and fifth decade. The commonest sites are the lower leg in females and the back in males but any body site, covered or uncovered may be involved.

In the early stages the SSMM may be very small (Figure 5.4) but the history of change and the irregular colour and outline are characteristic. As growth continues, the lesion spreads horizontally but may also become palpable with a central nodule suggesting progression to vertical growth phase. This represents a nodule arising in an SSMM rather than an NM. The differential diagnosis at this stage is usually between early MM or benign, atypical or dysplastic naevus. Benign melanocytic naevi vary considerably in appearance as they mature. The early, flat or slightly raised, brown junctional naevus often found in children and young adults may show

some variation in pigment which is often darker centrally. More mature compound naevi can be quite raised or papillomatous and range in colour from pale brown to almost black, although they are usually uniformly coloured. A noticeable increase in size and pigmentation may occur around puberty giving rise to family concern. Other differential diagnoses of SSMM include flat seborrhoeic wart, solar lentigo and pigmented actinic keratosis. On the face it can be particularly difficult to differentiate these lesions and biopsy may be required.

Nodular melanoma

Nodular melanoma is commoner in males, presenting usually in the fifth or sixth decade. The trunk is a common site. The tumours have no radial growth phase, invading vertically from the outset, so they are usually thick with a corresponding poor prognosis by the time they are removed (Figure 5.5). Clinically the tumour appears as a raised dome or nodule

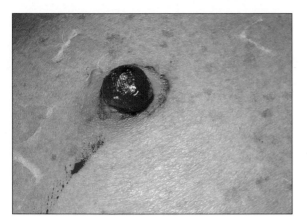

Figure 5.6
Amelanotic nodular melanoma arising in a naevus.

and is black-brown or reddish brown in colour. Rapid growth may lead to loss of pigmentation and an amelanotic tumour (Figure 5.6). Ulceration and bleeding are common in NM.

The differential diagnosis of NM includes benign Spitz naevus, pigmented basal cell carcinoma (BCC), dermatofibroma, angioma and traumatized seborrhoeic keratosis. Spitz naevus may be reddish brown or black and is a likely diagnosis in children. In pigmented BCC the history is of a slowly enlarging lesion and the pearly border is often discernible. Dermatofibromas are usually very firm in texture with a surrounding brown ring of haemosiderin staining. The dermatofibroma typically causes tethering of the overlying epidermis. Haemangiomas are often purple black in colour and may enlarge rapidly and bleed, leading to confusion with NM. Fleshy darkly pigmented seborrhoeic keratosis may mimic NM (and vice versa) particularly if the lesion is traumatized. Most dermatologists have at some time curetted off a 'seborrhoeic wart' only to find later that histology shows

MM and many seborrhoeic warts have been widely excised as 'MM', often by surgeons.

Lentigo maligna melanoma

This type of MM occurs as a late development in lentigo maligna (Hutchinson's melanotic freckle) which is the often-prolonged, in-situ or horizontal growth phase. Lentigo maligna melanoma occurs on exposed sites mostly on the face in older patients. The preceding lentigo maligna is a flat, brown or black macule, irregular in outline and pigmentation which grows very slowly, compared to SSMM. It may be many years before an invasive nodule develops indicating progression to vertical growth phase. When examining lentigo maligna, a Wood's light may be useful to demonstrate lateral extension of the lesion which may be imperceptible in ordinary light.

The differential diagnosis includes flat seborrhoeic keratosis and pigmented actinic keratosis. Both these benign lesions tend to have a dull, velvety or textured surface with some surface scaling. Solar or simple lentigo may also be confused in the early stages of lentigo maligna.

Acral lentiginous melanoma

In the white-skinned population this accounts for only 10% of MMs but it is the commonest MM in nonwhite-skinned races. 'Acral' skin is the thickened skin of the palms and soles and this type of MM comprises a flat lentiginous area usually on the sole but occasionally on the palm, with an invasive nodular component (Figure 5.7). The differential diagnosis includes benign naevus, haemorrhagic wart and black heel (talon noir) which is caused by haemorrhage into the epidermis.

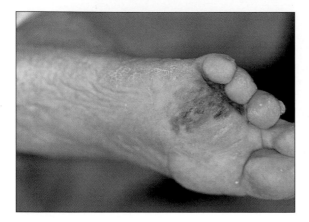

Figure 5.7
Acral lentiginous melanoma.

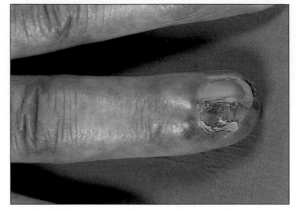

Figure 5.8
Subungual melanoma damaging the nailplate and showing Hutchinson's sign.

Subungual MM is a rare type of MM, which is often diagnosed late because of confusion with benign subungual naevus, traumatic haemorrhage, fungal infection or even subungual wart. Spillage of pigment onto the surrounding nailfold (Hutchinson's sign) is a strong indicator of malignancy (Figure 5.8). As the MM advances, the nail may be destroyed.

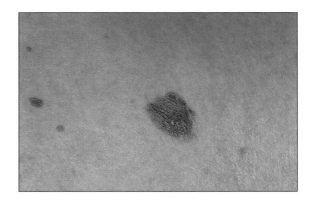

Figure 5.9
Early lesion of amelanotic melanoma (tiny speck of pigment may help with the diagnosis).

Amelanotic melanoma

The diagnosis of amelanotic MM is often missed clinically, coming to light only with the histology report. Flatter early lesions may be misdiagnosed as dermatitis, Spitz naevus, Bowen's disease or superficial BCC (Figure 5.9). Later nodular lesions may appear sinister on presentation with a history of rapid enlargement, bleeding and oozing of a nodular tumour. They may be mistaken for SCC or a secondary deposit or even rare entities such as a Merkel cell tumour. The lack of pigmentation is due to the rapid growth of the tumour and the dedifferentiation of the malignant melanocytes. Amelanotic MM has a similar natural history to its pigmented counterpart but delayed diagnosis is common, so that amelanotic tumours tend to be diagnosed at a more advanced stage and have a correspondingly poorer prognosis.

Pathology

Cytological and architectural features are important in the diagnosis of MM.

Symmetry

Whereas small symmetrical tumours are usually benign, the opposite is the case for most large, irregular and asymmetric lesions. Architectural asymmetry can relate to overall shape, lateral extensions, dermal extensions, lymphocytic infiltrate, epidermal involvement or pattern of pigmentation. Most benign lesions, with the exception of Spitz naevi and some dysplastic naevi, have a sharp lateral cut-off. Most melanoma have an indistinct lateral border with pagetoid spread of melanocytes.

Upward movement of melanocytes

The normal position for melanocytes is at the dermo-epidermal junction but in MM it is common for them to be seen at all levels of the epidermis, usually as single cells. The same pattern is occasionally also seen in Spitz naevus, recurrent naevus and congenital naevus of early infancy. When clumps or nests of cells are seen high in the epidermis it is usually a benign process and part of trans-epithelial elimination of these cells.

Intradermal component

Melanoma tend to demonstrate an irregular intradermal pattern. Areas of dense cellular grouping will be interspersed with sheets of diffuse tumour cells or a fibrotic stroma with inflammatory cells. Maturation, which is a tendency for smaller, fusiform cells to be seen towards the base is less common. An increased number of mitoses and nuclear atypia can be expected.

Reactive changes

There is usually a lymphocytic infiltrate with some fibrosis and angiogenesis irregularly distributed at the base of the tumour. Reactive epidermal hyperplasia may also be seen.

The pathologist's report

There has recently been agreement about which features should be included in the report (Table 5.2). This establishes the diagnosis,

Table 5.2
Elements of the pathologist's report.

Macroscopic
　　Full description of macroscopic appearance
　　Dimensions of the specimen
　　Dimensions of the lesion

Microscopic
　　Breslow thickness
　　Clarke level
　　Growth phase (radial or vertical)
　　Completeness of excision and measurement of margins

Other features which may affect prognosis
　　Features of regression
　　Vascular, lymphatic or neural invasion
　　Degree of lymphocytic invasion (absent, brisk and nonbrisk)
　　Presence or absence of ulceration
　　Presence of microsatellites
　　Mitotic activity

allows the proper treatment to be planned and helps to assess prognosis. The report should attempt to define whether it is a primary lesion, local recurrence or metastasis.

Factors predictive of metastasis and prognosis

In 1953 Allen and Spitz published a paper addressing the histological and clinical features which affected survival. There has been surprisingly little added to their work but gradually new data have helped to give increasingly accurate prognostic tables.

Clinical variables

Site is important and lesions on the extremities are less aggressive (except for those on the palm and soles) than those on the trunk, head and neck. The scalp is a particularly poor area. Malignant melanoma is more common on the back in men and the lower leg in women.

Some of the factors which give women a better prognosis may be due to the sites which are affected and the earlier stage at which they present to doctors. Younger women appear to do better than either men at any age or women over 50.

Histological variables

While the abnormal proliferation of melanocytes is entirely within the epidermis there is no potential for metastasis but when a vertical growth phase develops so does the risk of distant spread. The Breslow thickness is the single most important prognostic variable.

Table 5.3
Eight-year survival probability (tumours > 1.7 mm, no regression, lymphocytic response nonbrisk, on extremities).

Mitotic rate	Women	Men
0.0	0.98	0.95
0.1–6.0	0.95	0.86
> 6.0	0.84	0.63

There is a continuous linear association. Division of tumours into thickness subsets is for convenience. The level of dermal invasion may be an independent factor.

High mitotic rate is an important predictor of poor outcome. Ulceration of the tumour surface is also a high-risk factor but may be due, in part, to its association with high mitotic rate. A brisk lymphocytic inflammatory response is associated with a better prognosis. Finally there is some evidence that regression is linked to a poorer outcome. Typical 5-year disease-free survival for tumours of Breslow thickness less than 1.5 mm is 92% and for those greater than 3.5 mm it is 36%. An example of the relative importance of one other variable is summarized in Table 5.3.

Diagnostic methods

High-resolution ultrasound

The search continues for methods which will help to differentiate benign lesions from MM. Recent work using high-resolution ultrasound has shown promise in differentiating between seborrhoeic keratosis and MM. It was less able to distinguish between benign naevi and MM. Currently this is more likely to be useful to GPs than hospital specialists.

Clinical awareness

A clinical diagnosis is the basis for successful management of MM, but this may be more difficult than it sounds. Melanoma can be very difficult to detect by 'spot diagnosis', and when mistakes are made it is usually because all of the available clinical information has not been integrated to produce a sensible conclusion. Two case histories illustrate this important point.

A 29 year old woman has a 12-month history of a steadily enlarging but asymptomatic pigmented lesion on the skin of her leg. This has developed from previously normal skin, is 8 × 6 mm, and looks like a mid-brown seborrhoeic wart. However, seborrhoeic warts do not normally grow on the legs of young women, and do not normally grow to that size that quickly. We know that melanoma is commonest on the lower limb in females, that the age group 20 and upwards are at risk, that they can appear on previously normal skin without a precursor mole, and that early or thin melanoma can be very difficult to distinguish visually from benign lesions such as compound naevi or seborrhoeic warts. The lesion is excised, and is a superficial spreading melanoma, 0.7 mm in thickness.

A 75 year old man has a 5 mm diameter lesion on the nose with pale brown pigment that looks just like an intradermal naevus. However, he is adamant that it has only been present for 9 months, having arisen on normal skin, whereas intradermal naevi have a much longer history because they evolve over the years from junctional and then compound naevi. Although intradermal naevi do sometimes enlarge over a few months, this is unlikely to occur in a 75 year old. Excision showed a 2.3 mm thick nodular melanoma.

In both these patients the diagnosis was made because the history simply did not fit with the appearance, and this inconsistency led to the lesion being excised. Although the visual characteristics of MM can overlap with benign skin lesions, there are usually clues in the history, or the overall clinical picture, to indicate that the lesion might be malignant.

Biopsy technique

Another source of diagnostic error is biopsy technique. An incisional biopsy is not appropriate. The entire lesion should be excised with a 2 mm margin of clinically normal skin, including a layer of subdermal fat. There are two main reasons for this. The first is that incision biopsies are prone to sampling error. Melanomas often contain bits of benign or atypical moles, and if this is the area that is biopsied it could result in an incorrect diagnosis. Second, the overall appearance of the lesion is important: Is it symmetrical? Does it mature as it goes deeper? A biopsy may not allow this assessment. Third, treatment margins depend on accurate microstaging. This requires step sectioning of the entire lesion – it cannot reliably be predicted clinically, which is only a rough guide. Large lesions that cannot be closed primarily are best excised and left open until diagnosis and microstaging have been achieved and treatment can be planned. Incisional biopsy may rarely be justified for the palms and soles and subungual lesions. Also where a pigmented lesion is thought to be nonmelanocytic it may be best to confirm this histologically. There is rarely a place for incisional biopsy in primary care.

In a typical biopsy the direction of the ellipse should follow the relaxed skin tension lines and the skin excised with a 2 mm margin and down to subdermal fat. The longitudinal margin should be measured too. A marker suture may be useful for orientation if there is unsuspected adjacent subclinical disease on one side of the ellipse. Neat surgery is essential – approximately one in four biopsies in screening clinics will prove to be MM and the 75% of patients who do not require further treatment will not appreciate a nasty scar. Patients with MM are likely to find treatment easier to contemplate if their biopsy site has healed well and looks good.

There is no evidence that excision biopsy in any way adversely affects outcome, and it is impossible to rationally plan treatment without confirmation of the diagnosis and microstaging.

Explanation to the patient

It usually takes about 1 week to complete histopathology. However because it is a difficult area of histological diagnosis, up to 15% of lesions may require further pathological opinions. Facts that need to be available are the thickness of the tumour (in mm), the level of invasion, whether vascular invasion or local metastasis have occurred and the completeness of excision.

These facts allow the doctor to break the bad news with a clear explanation of what is wrong. The patient must be told that it is MM and in the case of in-situ lesions be told that cure can be certain – it is of course crucial that the entire lesion has been looked at by serial sections.

If the lesion is invasive the patient must be told that it can spread to local nodes or distant sites. This is modified according to risk. If the MM is a 0.5 mm thick level 2 lesion on the lower leg in a female, chance of cure is well over 95%. If it is a 2.8 mm level 4 lesion on the upper back of a male, chance of cure is much less, at around 60–65%. It is important to be honest, but realistically positive. Many patients with apparently awful disease will never have another problem, and they do not need a hopelessly negative portrayal of their situation at the time of diagnosis.

It is a good idea not to conduct the interview alone. Patients need continuing support following diagnosis, and this is best provided by a member of the nursing team preferably one who has already met the patient and who is experienced in nursing patients with MM.

Management (see Chapters 7–9 for details of surgical technique and adjuvant therapy and Appendix IV for British Association of Dermatologists guidelines)

Prevention

This is dealt with in Chapter 10.

Treatment

The treatment of primary MM, whether in situ or invasive, is surgical excision. A diagnostic procedure aims to completely remove the lesion to allow accurate diagnosis and microstaging. Treatment aims to minimize risk of local in-situ or invasive recurrence or metastasis due to incomplete removal of the primary, and risk of local metastasis due to incomplete removal of local subclinical metastatic disease.

Margins

For years the surgery of primary MM was mired in dogma. Surgical practice was to excise the tumour down to or including muscle fascia, frequently without a preceding excision biopsy to confirm the diagnosis, with very large margins of normal surrounding skin. The justification for this was the observed propensity for MM to metastasize to the skin and subcutaneous tissues in and around the primary site, so-called local recurrence or local metastasis. There was no agreed definition of this term – each study provided its own. In the UK the standard margin in the postwar years was 2 inches or 5 cm, but in the 1960s up to 15 cm had been recommended. As it became apparent that MM under 0.75 mm were very unlikely to metastasize, so the dogma of wide excision began to be challenged. The WHO Melanoma Group carried out the first randomized controlled trial of excision margins, comparing 3 cm with 1 cm margins in MMs up to 2 mm thick. Their first report, in 1988, appeared to show little difference in outcomes. However, there was a difference, which gradually became more apparent with longer follow-up. Only one MM had recurred locally (although the study does not define local recurrence) as the first site of relapse in the 3 cm group, whereas this had affected three patients in the 1 cm group. All had MMs in the thickness band 1–2 mm. Three years after the initial report this difference had increased to one and five, then one and six, and in 1993 was three and eight. In other words, it does seem that 1 cm margins are associated with a higher risk of local metastasis as first site of relapse than are 3 cm

margins. There are three possible explanations: the difference is either due to chance, to more aggressive disease or to less effective treatment. If increased risk of local metastasis simply reflects more aggressive disease, then it is unlikely that more aggressive local surgery will improve survival. If, however, it reflects bad treatment, it may matter. In this case it could mean that a narrow margin of excision had failed to remove local subclinical metastasis. If this was present without there being disease elsewhere, it would represent a missed opportunity for cure.

There is evidence in breast cancer that the extent of local treatment can affect survival, and so it is a reasonable idea that it might in MM. The question may be answered by the UK trial of 1 and 3 cm margins in MMs 2 mm and more in thickness which will first report in the next 2–3 years, but will then require a much longer follow-up. What are the surgical margins to use now to treat MM?

As well as the WHO trial, there are three further randomized trials, but only one of these provides useful extra information. The Intergroup trial investigated outcomes in MM of 1–4 mm treated with 2 or 4 cm margins. Outcomes were no different in the 2 cm group from the 4 cm group. However, there were so few patients in the 2–4 mm band that no firm conclusion can be drawn about the safety of a 2 cm margin. However, it appears to be safe for patients with MMs up to 2 mm in thickness.

The margins currently recommended are shown in Table 5.4. It is important to emphasize that there is not universal agreement about the best margins and as further studies are completed the strength of evidence will change. The 5–10 mm margin for in-situ MM is not based on evidence, but on the recommendation of a National Institutes of Health Consensus Group meeting held in 1992. Interestingly, a long-term follow-up study has

Table 5.4
Excision margins for melanoma.

Breslow depth (mm)	Minimum margin	Approx. 5 year survival
In situ	2–5 mm clinical margins to achieve complete histological excision	95–100%
< 1.0 mm	1 cm (narrower margins are probably safe in lesions <0.75 mm depth)	95–100%
1–2 mm	1–2 cm	80–96%
2.1–4 mm	2–3 cm (2 cm preferred)	60–75%
> 4 mm	2–3 cm	50%

Margins are clinically measured at surgery.

shown a 2 mm margin to be apparently adequate for some very thin MMs. Equally 2 mm margins have been used to treat in-situ melanoma of the lentigo maligna type, with a local in-situ recurrence rate of less than 5%. However in-situ and very thin MMs undoubtedly can recur within the scar, sometimes with invasive disease, following apparently complete excision with narrow margins. This approach cannot be recommended until there is more information about its efficacy.

All excisions for invasive MM should be down to, but not include, muscle fascia where present, since all of the published data on outcomes have used this deep surgical margin. Possible exceptions may be where the skin and subcutaneous fat are thin, and the MM is thick, for example, on the scalp, forehead, inner arm and dorsum of hand/foot.

Nearly all MM therapeutic excisions can be carried out under local anaesthesia. The exceptions are listed below.

- Lesions on the soles and palms, where infiltration anaesthesia is painful. These are best treated with, for example, ankle or sciatic nerve block, or general anaesthesia.

- Sites such as the buttock, where the thickness of subcutaneous fat may make infiltration anaesthesia difficult, especially in the obese.
- Ano-genital or other mucosal primaries.
- Primaries > 2 mm immediately adjacent to or over a regional lymph node basin. This is the only situation where a case might be made for elective lymph node dissection when a sentinel node procedure is not available (see later).

Invasive primary MM on the digits can be treated by amputation through the proximal interphalangeal joint and occasionally the metatarso- or metacarpo-phalangeal joint, depending on position. Some surgeons prefer MID shaft amputation. Head and neck primaries are usually straightforward to treat under local anaesthesia.

It may not be possible to treat all lesions with these margins, for instance, an MM on the free margin of the eyelid or on the ear or an MM of 2 mm or more in thickness on the cheek or on the sole. At all of these sites a margin of 1, 2 or 3 cm could produce significant functional and/or cosmetic impairment. A compromise is to carry out a procedure that will allow a surgical margin as close as possible to that normally required without producing unacceptable cosmetic or functional impairment. Defining the optimum procedure is usually a multidisciplinary decision.

The excision and repair (see Chapters 7 and 8)

The skin is incised to fat and then fascia, periosteum or muscle using blunt dissection where necessary to avoid named vessels and nerve trunks. A marker suture is placed in the specimen, and it is sent for histology. Direct closure is the preferred method, with layered closure with subcuticular vicryl, and subcuticular prolene where possible. Split skin grafts, preferably in unmeshed sheets, are the main alternative. Flaps, and to a lesser extent full thickness grafts, are used mainly on the head and neck, although full thickness grafts can produce surprisingly good results elsewhere.

Much of this surgery can be done in an outpatient setting. Frail, elderly patients, and those requiring larger excisions and grafts may require a short admission. Re-excision histology should confirm absence of both residual primary MM within the previous wound, and local metastatic disease. Despite preoperative counselling patients often think that negative re-excision histology means that the cancer has not spread, and that they are cured. It may be necessary to further discuss prognosis at this point.

Lymph nodes (sentinel node)

The question of lymph node dissection has vexed clinicians for a long time. Just as surgery for the primary lesion has become more conservative over the last 20 years so has surgery for possible lymph node involvement. Elective dissection of the nearest draining nodal basin is no longer common practice. There is now good evidence to show that it does not improve prognosis. Inevitably, however, some patients will have nodal metastases that cannot be detected clinically and we do not know why elective dissection in this group does not improve prognosis. There is nevertheless a strong feeling that if we could identify this group of patients it may be possible to treat them selectively with adjuvant therapy and enhance survival. Hence the concept of the sentinel node (SLN) biopsy.

The SLN is the first lymph node that a metastasis will encounter in the nodal basin draining the area of the MM. It is thought that MM spreads in an orderly fashion through lymph vessels to the SLN and then to more proximal nodes. Skip metastases, where a proximal node is involved but not the SLN, occur in less than 2% of patients. Blue dye or a radiolabelled agent is injected, intraoperatively, around the site of the tumour and the SLN identified by the uptake of dye or radioactivity. The gland is excised and one of several techniques used to detect micrometastases. If tumour is identified a dissection of the nodal basin or adjuvant therapy could be offered. Avoidance of further surgery and reassurance of the patient are two advantages that follow a negative investigation. Currently however there is no evidence that further surgery or adjuvant therapy, in the SLN positive group, confers any survival advantage. The morbidity of SLN biopsy and block dissection of nodes should not be underestimated. Currently SLN biopsy is a research tool for studying MM.

Laboratory tests and imaging
(Staging – see Table 5.5)

These investigations are done to discover those asymptomatic metastases for which an intervention might prolong life or reduce morbidity.

Table 5.5
AJCC/UICC staging system.

Stage	Primary tumour (pT)	Lymph node (N)	Distant metastases (M)
0	In situ tumours	No nodes	None
IA	<1.0 mm, no ulceration	No nodes	None
IB	<1.0 mm with ulceration	No nodes	None
	1.01–2.0 mm no ulceration	No nodes	None
IIA	1.01–2.0 mm with ulceration	No nodes	None
	2.01–4.0 mm no ulceration	No nodes	None
IIB	2.01–4.0 mm with ulceration	No nodes	None
	>4.0 mm no ulceration	No nodes	None
IIC	>4.0 mm with ulceration	No nodes	None
IIIA	Any Breslow thickness, no ulceration	Micrometastases in nodes	None
IIIB	Any Breslow thickness with ulceration	Micrometastases in nodes Up to 3 palpable nodes	None
	Any Breslow thickness, no ulceration	No nodes but in transit metastases or satellites	None
	Any Breslow thickness +/– ulceration		None
IIIC	Any Breslow thickness with ulceration	Up to 3 palpable nodes	None
	Any Breslow thickness +/– ulceration	Four or more palpable nodes or matted nodes or in transit metastases with nodes	None
IV	Any Breslow thickness		M1: skin, subcutaneous or distant lymph nodes M2: lung M3: all other sites or any site with raised lactate dehydrogenase

Apart from the cost of the investigation it may lead to further cost from additional work up or therapy. In 1992 an MM consensus workshop concluded that for MM < 1 mm thick no work up was indicated. Several workshops in Europe looked at stage I melanoma (that is, up to 1.5 mm) and recommended some blood tests and a baseline chest radiograph. Full blood count, lactate dehydrogenase and chest radiograph seems to be the most that is required in asymptomatic stage IB-3 patients. It is of interest that two retrospective reports on the detection of metastases showed that in stage I-3 MM, 95% of recurrent disease was identified by the history or physical examination. A further study on 145 asymptomatic patients with stage I–3 disease revealed that although all of them had a baseline CT scan of chest and abdomen/pelvis this failed to identify any of the 35 patients who went on to develop metastases or any of the seven who later developed regional nodal recurrence. If physical examination or history suggests metastatic disease then specific tests can be organized. CT of the chest is indicated if there is cervical or axillary adenopathy and CT of the pelvis if there is inguinal adenopathy.

Serological markers

Another approach to the problem of identifying patients who would most benefit from adjuvant therapy is to look for serological markers of disease either at the time of diagnosis, immediately after treatment of the primary tumour or at intervals during the entire period of follow-up. S100 protein, cytokines and their receptors, cell adhesion molecules and several other serological markers are more easily detected in the advanced stages of the disease. However, they are not sensitive markers so they cannot be used in staging procedures. Work is ongoing to find markers which might be useful in the early stages of disease or in the prediction of therapy outcome.

Follow-up

There is no general agreement on follow-up policy for patients with MM. Most specialists follow those with thin MM less frequently and for a shorter time but almost everyone will be seen at intervals for a year and in some centres up to 5 years. For intermediate thickness tumours most centres keep patients under review for 3–5 years and in some cases up to 10 years. For thick tumours the norm is probably 5–10 years or indefinitely in some centres. Usually follow-up is purely on clinical grounds but research or audit may be factors.

The reasons for follow-up change as time elapses following surgery. Initially there is a healing wound to review which, after a wide excision, may be deep or involve a flap or graft. Patients often need reassurance about other moles they have noticed and a range of vague symptoms for which there is rarely an organic basis. It is also a time to discuss prognosis, new treatments, lifestyle and the psychological aspects of the disease. A physical examination, with the patient in underwear, allows assessment of the entire skin surface for other pigmented lesions. The surgical scar, all lymph nodes and an abdominal palpation complete the routine. Many specialists now encourage the patient to learn self-examination of lymph nodes. Just as breast or testicular self-examination are acceptable to most people so lymph nodes can be assessed regularly by the melanoma patient. They are the most likely site of spread and by no means all node involvement is picked up at a routine follow-up visit.

A recent audit of practices in a four-manned subregional plastic surgery unit highlighted not only the differences between each surgeon but also the noncompliance of each team with the unit's policy. Harmonization of the four policies not only led to improved compliance by 54% but also reduced clinic costs.[8]

References

1. MacKie RM, Hole D et al (1997) Cutaneous malignant melanoma in Scotland: incidence, survival, and mortality, 1979–94, *Br Med J* 315:1117–21.
2. Esterly NB (1996) Management of congenital melanocytic naevi: a decade later, *Pediatr Dermatol* 13:321–40.

3. Castilla EE, de Graca M, Orioli-Parreiras IM (1981) Epidemiology of congenital pigmented naevi: incidence rates and relative frequencies, *Br J Dermatol* **104**:307–15.
4. MacKie RM, English J, Aitchison TC et al (1985) The number and distribution of benign pigmented moles (melanocytic naevi) in a healthy British population, *Br J Dermatol* **113**:167–74.
5. Consensus Conference on Precursors to Malignant Melanoma (1985) *J Dermatol Surg Oncol* **11**:537–42.
6. Swerdlow AJ, Weinstock MA (1998) Do tanning lamps cause melanoma? An epidemiologic assessment, *J Am Acad Dermatol* **38**:89–98.
7. Kraemer KH, Greene MH, Tarone R et al (1983) Dysplastic naevi and cutaneous melanoma risk, *Lancet* **ii**(8358):1076–7.
8. Hormbrey E, Banwell P, Gillespie P et al (2000) Melanoma follow-up; protocols and practice, *Br J Dermatol* **142**:585.

Bibliography

Easton D (1996) The role of atypical mole syndrome and cutaneous naevi in the development of melanoma, *Cancer Surv* **26**:237–48.

MacKie RM (1998) Incidence, risk factors and prevention of melanoma, *Eur J Cancer* **34**(Suppl 3):S3–6.

Kirkham N, Cotton OWK, Lallemand RC et al (eds) (1992) *Diagnosis and Management of Melanoma in Clinical Practice* (Springer: Berlin).

Huang CL et al (1998) Laboratory tests and imaging studies in patients with cutaneous malignant melanoma, *J Am Acad Dermatol* **39**:451–63.

6 Rare skin tumours and metastatic disease

Clinicians dealing with skin cancer are sometimes confronted with atypical lesions where a clinical diagnosis is not possible. The differential diagnosis should include not only the three commonest tumours, with unusual presenting features, but also rarer tumours of epidermal origin. Metastatic deposits in the skin can normally be differentiated from primary skin tumours because they tend to be dermal but this is not always easy and if ulceration has occurred it may become impossible. This chapter deals with other tumours of epidermal origin and tumours which have metastasized to the skin.

Rare skin tumours

Tumours of epidermal origin

Verrucous carcinoma

Verrucous carcinoma is a rare low-grade squamous cell carcinoma (SCC) of skin and mucous membrane, which carries a favourable prognosis. Clinically the tumour appears as an exuberant mass, which invades locally but rarely metastasizes. There appears to be a link between human papilloma virus infection and the development of some verrucous carcinoma. Histologically all verrucous carcinomas are well-differentiated SCCs, rarely showing dysplastic features. All types are more common in the male. There are four types of verrucous carcinoma based on their anatomical site.

- Giant condyloma acuminata (Buschke–Lowenstein tumour). Seen in the anogenital region, often on the uncircumcised penis, developing as a large warty lesion which slowly spreads over penis and scrotum.
- Ackerman tumour. Found in the oropharynx appearing as a florid papillomatosis on a background of leucoplakia. Heavy alcohol intake and chewing of tobacco or betel predispose to this tumour.
- Carcinoma cuniculatum. A warty tumour on the sole of the foot and rarely the palm often mistaken for a verruca which resists all treatment. It slowly burrows into the underlying soft tissue and even bone with areas of ulceration and hyperkeratosis progressing to a malodorous cauliflower-like mass.
- Cutaneous verrucous carcinoma. This refers to lesions in all other sites, for example, face, scalp, trunk and limbs. It may develop in chronic ulcers or scars.

Management of verrucous carcinoma is usually surgical by wide local excision possibly with Mohs' micrographic surgery. Carbon dioxide laser surgery has been advocated and photodynamic therapy has been used for vulval and laryngeal verrucous carcinoma. Treatment with bleomycin, etretinate and intralesional interferon have all been described as adjuvant therapy. The role of radiotherapy is controversial as there have been reported cases of anaplastic change in verrucous carcinomas following treatment. However some cases have responded well to radiotherapy.

Tumours of epidermal appendages

Appendageal or adnexal tumours arise from the pilosebaceous unit, the apocrine and eccrine glands. The pilosebaceous units are concentrated in the skin of the head, neck and upper trunk so tumours arising from these structures will be found mainly at these sites. Eccrine glands are located all over the body including the palms. The great majority of tumours derived from epidermal appendages are benign. Malignant tumours are rare and the appearance of most of these tumours is nonspecific so that the diagnosis is usually made histologically after biopsy.

Sebaceous carcinoma

This malignant tumour shows differentiation towards sebaceous epithelium. About 75% of sebaceous carcinoma are periocular where it is also known as meibomian gland carcinoma. Most of these are seen on the upper eyelid of elderly patients. Clinically it appears as a firm, slowly enlarging nodule resembling a chalazion but sometimes it may mimic an inflammatory condition such as blepharoconjunctivitis and diagnosis may be delayed. Extra-ocular sebaceous carcinoma usually

occurs on the face or scalp as a very slowly enlarging nodule, which may reach many centimetres in size without metastasizing. There is an association with Torre–Muir syndrome (a cancer-associated genodermatosis) and 25% of patients with Torre–Muir syndrome develop sebaceous carcinoma. Prior radiotherapy and arsenic ingestion have also been associated with the development of sebaceous carcinoma.

It is an aggressive tumour with a poor prognosis due to its high recurrence rate and tendency to metastasize widely. Local recurrence after surgery occurs in up to 36% of cases. Metastasis occurs by lymphatic or haematogenous spread or by direct invasion of the lacrimal system. Poor prognosis is indicated by ocular location, multifocal origin, poor differentiation and infiltrative growth pattern, with an overall 5-year survival of 30%. Complete resection by wide local excision or by Mohs' micrographic surgery with margin control is indicated. Postoperative adjuvant radiotherapy may be advised.

Eccrine carcinoma

Malignant tumours of sweat glands are rare. Some occur when malignant change develops in a pre-existing benign lesion such as an eccrine poroma. These tend to behave in a relatively benign manner and rarely metastasize. Others develop as carcinomas from the outset and may behave more aggressively with a propensity to metastasize. There are a number of malignant tumours of eccrine sweat gland origin with distinctive histological or clinical features.

'Classic' sweat gland carcinoma: This may be of eccrine, or less commonly apocrine origin, occurring in both sexes in later life. The tumour appears as a slowly enlarging, reddish or purple nodule, which is firm, sometimes tender and lobular. They occur anywhere including the palm but are more common on the head and neck. Metastasis is frequent via lymphatic spread and distant metastases may show epidermotropism, invading distant epidermis. Wide local excision is required and radical surgery may be indicated for regional lymphatic spread.

Microcystic adnexal carcinoma (sclerosing sweat duct carcinoma): This tumour appears as a slowly enlarging indurated plaque on the central face of young or middle-aged individuals, more commonly males. There may be sensory changes secondary to perineural invasion. Wide excision ideally with micrographic surgery to identify and eradicate perineural invasion is recommended, particularly as these patients are often young. Metastasis is rare but recurrent disease requires aggressive surgery.

Eccrine epithelioma (basal cell carcinoma with eccrine differentiation): This rare tumour with clusters of basaloid cells in a dense stroma often extends into subcutaneous fat. It appears as a nonspecific tumour in the scalp and large lesions may ulcerate and cause pain. Wide excision is required (ideally with micrographic surgery) as local recurrence is common: metastasis is rare. Adjuvant radiotherapy may be beneficial.

Mucinous eccrine carcinoma: This rare tumour presents as a solitary, translucent, blue-grey cyst in middle-aged individuals. It is most common in the periorbital area and may appear similar to a benign hidrocystoma. Another important clinical differential diagnosis to consider is cutaneous secondary deposit from a common mucin-secreting tumour such as gastric carcinoma. Eccrine mucinous carcinoma follows an indolent course but occasional metastases have been reported. Wide excision, possibly with micrographic surgery, is recommended.

Adenoid cystic carcinoma (primary cutaneous adenocystic carcinoma): This is the rarest eccrine carcinoma and histologically resembles the relatively common adenoid cystic carcinoma of salivary gland origin. Primary cutaneous adenoid cystic carcinoma occurs as a nonspecific, sometimes painful nodule or plaque on the head or neck, with a predilection for the external auditory canal. Wide local excision is required, ideally with micrographic surgery which will allow for tissue conservation on the head and neck. Local recurrence is common after conventional surgery and metastasis to the lung has been recorded.

Extramammary Paget's disease

Extramammary Paget's disease (EMPD) is a rare intraepithelial adenocarcinoma, which may be associated with an underlying carcinoma such as rectum, urethra, cervix or bladder, or occasionally a distant carcinoma. It usually involves the anogenital region or the axillary folds. Rarely other locations can be involved such as eyelid, external ear, nose or chest.

The early clinical appearance shows a sharply demarcated erythematous plaque with a scaly or crusty surface, which may be eroded. Occasionally the surface may be papillomatous. Itching and burning occur early and may induce excoriation or lichenification. The eruption spreads relentlessly and is unresponsive to all topical applications customarily given (topical steroids, antibiotics, antifungals and emollients). The plaque extends very slowly and may evade diagnosis for many years. The differential diagnosis includes eczema, psoriasis and intertrigo but the inexorable course of EMPD is unlike the fluctuating pattern of these conditions. Lichen sclerosis et atrophicus needs to be considered in the anogenital region. Bowen's disease tends to be more raised and verrucous and superficial basal cell carcinoma usually demonstrates the typical pearly margin. Biopsy is conclusive.

The prognosis of EMPD varies, being more favourable if the histology shows the tumour is purely intraepithelial with no evidence of invasion. In 25% of cases there will be an underlying malignancy and the prognosis depends on the stage of that tumour. In perianal disease 33% have adenocarcinoma of the rectum and an associated mortality of 25%. Treatment of EMPD is usually surgical with wide local excision. More invasive EMPD requires wide and deep resection with lymph node dissection. There is a high recurrence rate following surgery and this is attributed to the multifocal nature of the condition and to the subclinical extension of tumour cells beyond the visible clinical margin. When EMPD is associated with an underlying carcinoma its recurrence rate is about 50%. Micrographic surgery offers better margin control. Photodynamic therapy has been reported to be successful in EMPD and may be particularly useful for invisible subclinical extension. Carbon dioxide laser treatment has also been used. Topical 5-fluorouracil cream may be used as an adjuvant to surgery but is only effective in noninvasive disease, confined to the epidermis. Radiotherapy has been used in patients who are unsuitable for surgery but adenocarcinoma generally responds poorly to radiation. Long-term follow-up is required.

Apocrine carcinoma

This is an exquisitely rare primary cutaneous adenocarcinoma arising in areas of greatest apocrine gland concentration. Thus the tumours occur most frequently in the axilla, external auditory canal, anogenital region, eyelid and breast. Clinically apocrine carcinoma appears as solitary or multiple nontender mobile subcutaneous nodules in middle-aged individuals. Previous radiotherapy may predispose to development of the tumour. The tumour is locally aggressive and in about 50% of cases metastasis occurs to regional lymph nodes. Surgery is the definitive treatment with wide local excision and regional lymph node dissection if indicated. The role of radiotherapy and chemotherapy is uncertain.

Tumours of muscle origin

Leiomyosarcoma

Primary leiomyosarcoma is a tumour of smooth muscle origin, which rarely affects skin. When it does so it develops from erector pili muscle while subcutaneous leiomyosarcoma arises from the media of large blood vessels. The distinction between cutaneous and subcutaneous leiomyosarcoma is important as the subcutaneous form carries a much poorer prognosis.

Leiomyosarcoma presents during the fifth to seventh decade. There is usually an asymptomatic nodule but pain has been reported. The surface epidermis of the lesion may show discolouration or umbilication. The differential diagnosis includes cyst, dermatofibroma, lipoma and neurofibroma but as it is such a rarity, it is seldom diagnosed prior to excision.

The prognosis for cutaneous disease tends to be good although local metastasis has rarely been reported. However subcutaneous leiomyosarcoma causes distant metastases in a third of patients, notably to lung and bone. Wide local excision with 3–5 cm margins or Mohs' micrographic surgery is advocated. Local recurrence rates of 40–60% are reported with cutaneous and subcutaneous leiomyosarcoma, usually within the first 5 years after surgery, and careful follow-up is required.

Tumours of adipose origin

Liposarcoma

Liposarcoma is a relatively common tumour which arises from the muscle fascia and extends into the subcutaneous fat. Rarely liposarcoma can originate from the subcutaneous fat itself but it is not thought to develop from a pre-existing lipoma. Clinically the tumour presents as an ill-defined nodular infiltrate on the lower extremities of a middle-aged individual. It is very rare in children and young adults. There are various histological subtypes of liposarcoma and the better-differentiated types carry the best prognosis with least chance of metastasis. Local recurrence occurs in 45–75% and metastases develop in 15–45%. Overall survival is 45–65% at 5 years and 20–50% at 10 years. Wide local excision followed by adjuvant radiotherapy is the treatment of choice for liposarcoma. Chemotherapy for metastases does not seem to alter the course of the disease.

Tumours of vascular origin

Angiosarcoma (malignant haemangioendothelioma)

Angiosarcoma is a rare malignant vascular tumour arising from both vascular and lymphatic endothelium. A rare form may affect children but the tumour is usually seen on the scalp or face of elderly individuals, men more frequently than women. Clinically the early lesion appears as a bruise-like purple or dusky red discoloration, which extends in area and slowly progresses to an infiltrated plaque which may ulcerate. In poorly differentiated tumours there may be swelling with a tumid appearance and rapid progression. The better-differentiated tumours advance more slowly but all carry an extremely poor prognosis. Rarely it appears in areas of chronic lymphoedema. The tumour characteristically invades and destroys locally and then metastasizes to both regional nodes and distant sites such as lung, liver and spleen. Mortality is more than 50% at 1 year and 5-year survival is less than 25%. The sizes of the lesion at presentation as well as the histological differentiation are important prognostic indicators. Smaller (< 5 cm), well-differentiated tumours carry a better prognosis. Combined surgery and radiotherapy are currently the best treatments available. Angiosarcoma usually extends well beyond the clinical margin so complete surgical resection is difficult to achieve. Preoperative tumour mapping by multiple biopsies around the perimeter of the lesion may improve the prospect of clearance. Following excision, adjuvant radiotherapy is recommended with wide field electron beam.

Tumours of neural origin

Merkel cell tumour (trabecular cell carcinoma, neuroendocrine carcinoma)

This is an aggressive cutaneous malignancy of neural origin, thought to derive from cutaneous Merkel cells. The normal Merkel cell is thought to be a secondary sensory cell acting as a mechanoreceptor and lying in the dermo-epidermal junction closely associated with nerve fibres. Merkel cell tumour presents as a rapidly growing, painless, red or violaceous nodule on sun-exposed skin in the elderly. Most Merkel cell tumours occur on the head and neck. The tumour is usually less than 2 cm but lesions up to 15 cm have been documented. The differential diagnosis includes squamous cell carcinoma, amelanotic melanoma, metastatic carcinoma deposit and keratoacanthoma, which may all enlarge rapidly. Basal cell carcinoma and epidermal cyst will develop more slowly. The diagnosis of Merkel cell tumour is rarely suspected prior to biopsy.

It is an aggressive tumour with a high local recurrence rate of 30% in the first year. Metastases to regional lymph nodes occur in more than half the patients and distant metastases to liver, bone, brain and lung ultimately occur in more than a third. Overall 5-year survival in Merkel cell carcinoma is around 50%. Aggressive wide local excision with a 2–3 cm margin is advised. This is often difficult as most lesions occur on the head and neck. Mohs' micrographic surgery with histological control of the margins is valuable in detecting and eradicating the deep extensions of Merkel cell carcinoma, which often penetrate into muscle. Merkel cell carcinoma appears to be radiosensitive and postoperative adjuvant radiotherapy has been advocated. Chemotherapy is used for regional and metastatic disease.

Tumours of fibrous origin

Dermatofibrosarcoma protuberans

Dermatofibrosarcoma protuberans (DFSP) is a low-grade, locally invasive tumour arising in the dermis from fibroblasts. It usually occurs in young or middle-aged individuals, rarely in children and has an equal sex distribution. Early lesions appear as one or more painless flesh coloured or red dermal nodules. Common locations include the trunk and proximal extremities but any area may be affected, including the head and neck. Progression is very slow. Long-standing lesions may eventually ulcerate and bleed and if neglected they may eventually invade deeper structures

including fascia, muscle and bone. The differential diagnosis in the early stages includes morphoea, keloid scar and dermatofibroma. The irregular, discoloured nodular plaque of the more advanced DFSP is usually distinctive.

Dermatofibrosarcoma protuberans is notorious for its tendency to recur after excision. While it is locally invasive, it rarely metastasizes and usually this occurs only after multiple local recurrences. Even after wide local excision with a 3 cm margin, a large series reported a recurrence rate of 20%. Mohs' micrographic surgery gives much improved results with 1.6% overall recurrence rate and this makes it the treatment of choice for DFSP, particularly as the risk of metastasis appears to be increased by repeated local excisions. If Mohs' surgery is not available, then a 5 cm margin down to and including fascia is recommended. The use of radiotherapy in DFSP is controversial. There are reports of high-grade malignant transformation of DFSP following radiotherapy used either as definitive or adjuvant therapy.

Cutaneous metastatic tumours

Cutaneous metastases are relatively uncommon, being seen in only 3% of primary neoplasms. However, important information for the diagnosis, prognosis and treatment of the primary cancer can be gained by properly evaluating these metastatic deposits.

Incidence

Most malignant tumours may spread to the skin. Certain cancers, notably renal cell carcinoma and malignant melanoma, appear to spread to the skin more frequently than would be expected from the incidence of the primary lesion. For most other cancers the incidence of cutaneous metastasis correlates with the incidence of the underlying primary tumour. Useful diagnostic information may accrue by considering the data collected by Brownstein and Helwig. They reviewed the data on 724 patients with cutaneous metastases, taking into account the patients' age, sex and site of the metastase, and described the following patterns.

Sex

In men the frequency of occurrence of metastasis from various tumours to the skin was carcinoma of the lung – 24%, carcinoma of the large bowel – 19%, malignant melanoma – 13% and SCC of the oral cavity – 12%. The pattern in women was strikingly different with carcinoma of the breast accounting for 69% of cases, carcinoma of the large bowel for 9% and melanoma, lung and ovary for only 4–5%.

Age

Malignant melanoma was more likely to be the cause of a cutaneous metastase in younger patients in both sexes. Over the age of 40 years, the pattern of occurrence by sex was enhanced, with 27% of cutaneous metastases arising from carcinoma of the lung in men, and in women carcinoma of the breast was the primary in over 72% of cases.

Site

In men most metastases are found on the head, neck, anterior chest and abdomen. This correlates with the commonest underlying primary,

that is, lung. Large bowel cancer spreads to the abdomen and pelvic region. Carcinoma of the oral cavity spreads to the face and neck. In women the localization is different and reflects the different incidence of primaries, the vast majority of metastatic tumours being found on the anterior chest as they arise from carcinoma of the breast.

Clinical features

The clinical form of the cutaneous metastases reflects the method of spread of the tumour. Cutaneous metastases from carcinoma of the breast provide good examples of the array of clinicopathological types of spread that are encountered.

Carcinoma of the breast

Breast cancer usually spreads directly along tissue plains or via lymphatics and thus produces a variety of clinical forms of cutaneous metastases.

Inflammatory carcinoma (carcinoma erysipeloides): This is due to the spread of malignant cells through the lymphatics of the dermis and subcutis. Involved skin is red and indurated with a well-demarcated edge like erysipelas.

Telangiectatic carcinoma (carcinoma telangiectoides): This results from spread in superficial lymphatics and dermal vessels. Clinically it may resemble a haemolymphangioma with telangiectatic nodules, plaques and vesicular areas.

Scirrhous carcinoma (cancer en cuirasse): It resembles a sclerotic plaque of morphoea. There is a marked fibrous stroma with a paucity of malignant cells. A similar form of metastasis to hair-bearing skin can lead to patchy hair loss termed alopecia neoplastica.

Peau d'orange: Lymphatic blockage by a neoplastic infiltrate may lead to localized lymphoedema which gives an appearance similar to orange peel.

Paget's disease of the nipple: If the tumour cells invade the epidermis directly, scaling, exudation and ulceration occur. This begins on the nipple or the skin of the areola and is always associated with an underlying cancer in that breast.

Carcinoma of the lung

Cutaneous metastases from a primary in the lung often spread haematogenously, thus they can be found in any skin site and often are apparent before the primary cancer has been recognized. Clinically they appear as firm nodules; although they may be single, multiple deposits often appear over a short time course.

Renal carcinoma

The cutaneous metastases from renal carcinoma are often diagnosed histologically before the primary tumour has become apparent. The metastases occur in all body sites, usually as an intradermal nodule with a marked vascular element.

Intra-abdominal tumours

Cutaneous metastases from cancer of the gastro-intestinal tract or the ovaries often develop on the abdominal wall. If the metastatic cells spread via the ligamentum teres the metastases will develop at the umbilicus – the so-called Sister Joseph's nodule.

Malignant melanoma

In approximately 5% of cases of metastatic melanoma found in the skin or subcutis no primary melanoma can be detected. The primary may have occurred on a nonexposed site such as the ano-rectal mucosa or it may be due to regression of the original primary. Melanoma may metastasize via the lymphatics or bloodstream. Lymphatic spread results in local or regional cutaneous metastases whereas haematogenous spread results in disseminated lesions. One curious feature following excision and grafting of a primary melanoma is the later occurrence of metastases within the graft donor site, especially if taken from the same limb as the primary tumour. It is recommended that if a skin graft is required to cover the excision site, that it is harvested from the contralateral limb.

Prognosis

The presence of cutaneous metastases invariably points to a poor prognosis as it indicates the advanced state of the malignant disease. Patients with multiple cutaneous metastases have a median survival time of 3 months.

Different primary tumours may develop their cutaneous metastases at different temporal points in the cancerous process. With breast cancer the primary tumour has usually been discovered prior to the development of the skin lesions. In contrast, in men with cancer of the lung or the kidney, half of the cutaneous metastases become apparent before the discovery of the primary tumour. In this situation histological examination of the cutaneous deposit will provide important diagnostic as well as prognostic information.

Treatment

Although the presence of cutaneous metastases indicates the dissemination of the malignant disease, occasionally solitary cutaneous deposits are found. Excision of a solitary metastasis and subsequent treatment of the primary tumour may dramatically improve the survival of patients in rare instances.

For the majority of patients excision of the cutaneous metastases is a palliative procedure. However as these metastases can enlarge rapidly and ulcerate it can greatly enhance the quality of life of a patient with a terminal disease. In addition the removal of the visible evidence of the underlying cancerous disease can provide comfort to those patients having difficulty in coming to terms with their malignant disease.

Bibliography

Brownstein MH and Helwig EB (1972) Patterns of cutaneous metastasis, *Arch Dermatol* **105**:862–8.

Schwartz RA (1995) Cutaneous metastatic disease, *J Am Acad Dermatol* **33**:161–82.

7 Treatment 1 – nonexcisional methods

In earlier chapters of this book aetiology, epidemiology and clinical aspects of skin cancer were emphasized. The principles of management were outlined including concepts such as margins of excision, dealing with recurrent or incompletely excised tumours and the appropriateness of different treatment modalities according to a variety of patient and tumour variables. Here and in Chapter 8 technical and theoretical aspects of the available treatments are discussed.

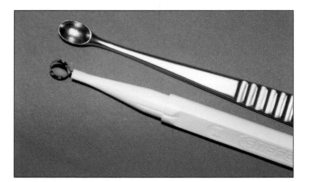

Figure 7.1
Spoon-shaped (Volkmann) and ring (Stiefel) curettes.

Curettage and cautery

Curettage is a technique commonly used in dermatological surgery for the removal of superficial lesions and it is performed under local anaesthesia. The curette is either an oval, semisharp, spoon-shaped instrument or an open ring connected to a handle (Figure 7.1). Different sizes allow the operator to deal with lesions which range from tiny papillomas to exophytic tumours several centimetres in diameter. The curette is designed to cut through abnormally soft or friable tissue with minimum force so that the diseased tissue can be selectively removed. The spoon-shaped variety is not as sharp and more easily finds a plane whereas the sharper, ring-shaped instrument is more likely to cut through normal tissue and must be handled with great care. A curette is held like a pencil, with the hand steadied on the patient, at a 20–45° angle to the surface of the skin. With the skin stretched and fixed by the other hand, the curette is then drawn towards the surgeon, gently scraping the lesion from the normal underlying skin. For larger lesions the curette can be gripped in the palm of the hand and used like a potato peeler, but fine control and sensation may be lost. The nature of this semisharp instrument allows the surgeon to feel the difference between normal and abnormal tissue such that curettage can be repeated until all abnormal tissue is removed. This is particularly useful when treating tumours because malignant tissue is usually softer and more friable than normal skin, enabling the surgeon to identify the margins of the tumour. The curetted material can be sent for pathological examination. Haemostasis is achieved by chemical cautery, electrocautery or diathermy and healing is relatively quick due to the superficial nature of this technique.

For the successful treatment of tumours, curettage is best used for primary, superficial, well-demarcated, nonfibrous, small tumours in low-risk areas and should be combined with subsequent electrocautery which destroys additional tissue. Two or three cycles of curettage and cautery have been advocated for the treatment of tumours. If the curette passes easily through the dermis into the subcutaneous fat, suggesting a deep tumour, curettage should be abandoned in favour of other treatment modalities.

If curettage is performed well complications are uncommon but include atrophy, hyper- or hypo-pigmentation, delayed healing and hypertrophic scarring.

Solar keratoses

These lesions are easily and effectively removed by curettage with an excellent cosmetic result. Curettage is less practicable and less well tolerated in patients with extensive disease. However it is useful when dealing with a small number of lesions and has the advantage of producing a specimen for pathological examination.

Bowen's disease

When Bowen's disease (BD) is treated by curettage and cautery the reported recurrence rate is around 20%. This relatively high rate may be due to the fact that lesions are often ill defined and may be larger than clinically evident. In addition, recurrence after curettage and electrodesiccation has been attributed to residual involvement of adnexal structures. In the treatment of erythroplasia of Queyrat, a recurrence rate of over 83% has been reported for light desiccation and curettage alone.[1]

Basal cell carcinoma

Different curettes and varying numbers of treatment cycles have been advocated. However good technique and careful patient selection are crucial for success. A large curette is used to scoop out the majority of the tumour and this piece is sent for histology. The edge and base are then scraped with a smaller instrument to try and remove residual pockets of tumour. With experience small extensions can be detected and extirpated. Most practitioners then cauterize a further rim of tissue all around before further scraping with the curette and finally achieving haemostasis. A review of published studies suggested an overall 5-year cure rate of 92.3% for primary basal cell carcinoma (BCC) and 60% for recurrent BCC.[2] The technique is best suited to small, well-defined, primary lesions in noncritical sites and with nonaggressive histology. It is generally not recommended for the management of large BCC, morphoeic BCC, recurrent tumours or those in the high-risk sites of nose, nasolabial fold and periorbital regions.

Experienced clinicians may use curettage combined with other modalities. In Chapter 3 its use to debulk a BCC, helping to delineate the clinical margins prior to excision, was discussed. Curettage and cryotherapy can be helpful together and are discussed later in this chapter.

Occasionally curettage is useful in the palliative management of extensive tumours.

In the very elderly, those restricted to bed or those with other significant medical problems it may be beneficial to debulk a large, exudative or malodorous tumour making their nursing care simpler.

Squamous cell carcinoma

The technique described for BCC is suitable for some squamous cell carcinomas (SCCs). Cure rates of 96–100% with 1–5 years follow-up have been reported.[3] Experience suggests that selecting small (< 1 cm), well-differentiated, primary slow-growing tumours ensures high cure rates.

Photodynamic therapy

Photodynamic therapy (PDT) uses the combination of a photosensitizer, which preferentially accumulates in malignant cells, and photoactivation by visible light to kill tumour cells.[4] Most clinical experience of PDT has been gained with the use of systemic haematoporphyrin derivatives. Unfortunately, the haematoporphyrin derivatives produce a generalized cutaneous photosensitivity lasting for up to 8–10 weeks after treatment which has severely limited their use in routine clinical practice.

5-Aminolaevulinic acid (ALA) PDT is a novel method which utilizes the haem synthesis pathway by which haem is produced from glycine and succinyl CoA. The administration of excess exogenous ALA results in a build-up of protoporphyrin IX (PpIX), the photosensitizer species responsible for the photodynamic effect. The topical application of ALA to solar keratoses, BD, SCC and BCC induces PpIX fluorescence and photosensitization that remains localized to the lesions, with much less fluorescence in adjacent normal skin and normal dermis. 5-Aminolaevulinic acid-induced PpIX fluorescence studies have confirmed a tumour:normal skin fluorescence ratio of up to 15:1. It is this tissue specificity that is thought to result in good healing and a very good cosmetic result.

Topical ALA is usually applied for 3–6 h under occlusion followed by irradiation by visible light. Lasers, producing red light around 630 nm, may be used for the photoactivation of photosensitizers used in PDT. However, narrow- or broadband nonlaser light sources, including modified slide projectors, have also been used effectively. Discomfort during irradiation, which is variable and unpredictable, may require local anaesthesia. Topical ALA PDT is a convenient, outpatient treatment in which multiple lesions can be treated simultaneously. There is no toxicity or interaction with other medications and healing and cosmetic results may be superior to conventional modalities. The lack of evidence for any cumulative toxicity or interaction with other treatment modalities makes it particularly helpful in the management of recurrent disease.

There is much work to be done to optimize current treatment parameters and combinations of photosensitizer and light source, whilst also developing new photosensitizers and light sources. In particular ALA esters are currently being developed to improve depth of penetration and distribution of photosensitization.

Solar keratoses

The superficial nature of solar keratoses and the ability to treat large areas with a good cosmetic result suggest that topical ALA PDT may be a useful treatment modality. Most

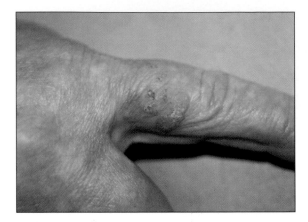

Figure 7.2
Patch of Bowen's disease before
photodynamic therapy.

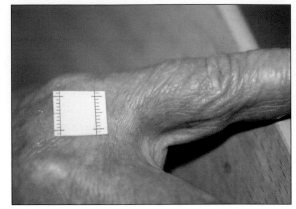

Figure 7.3
Same area as shown in Figure 7.2 following
successful photodynamic therapy.

clinical studies have reported a complete response rate of 80–100%. A single treatment appears to be as effective and as well tolerated as three weeks of twice daily topical 5-fluorouracil (5-FU) in the treatment of solar keratoses on the hands. Actinic cheilitis has also been successfully treated.

Bowen's disease

Systemic PDT with laser light irradiation was used to treat two patients with a total of over 500 lesions of BD and at follow-up 6 months later no lesions remained in either patient. Using topical ALA PDT complete response rates of 87–100% have been reported after a median follow-up of 12–24 months.[5] There is no delayed healing or ulceration and cosmesis is very good (Figures 7.2 and 7.3). In limited BD of the glans penis topical ALA PDT has also been shown to be effective. Specific destruction of hair follicles with resulting hair loss has been demonstrated with topical ALA PDT in animals and humans. The treatment

therefore offers tumour selectivity including involvement of skin appendages.

In a randomized, controlled study comparing topical ALA PDT with cryosurgery for the treatment of BD there was a complete response rate after 1 year of 90% in the cryosurgery group and 100% in the PDT group (not a statistically significant difference).[5] Ulceration occurred in 25% of lesions treated by cryosurgery but in none of the PDT-treated lesions. Topical ALA PDT appeared to be at least as effective as cryosurgery but with fewer adverse effects.

The excellent healing and final cosmetic result following PDT have in some centres made PDT the treatment of first choice for large patches of BD in elderly patients with fragile, atrophic and actinically damaged skin.[6]

Basal cell carcinoma

Complete response rates of 31–100% have been reported for the treatment of BCC using PDT with intravenously administered porphyrins. Using topical ALA PDT to treat superficial BCC, initial complete response rates of 88–100% have been reported, but with a subsequent recurrence rate of up to 38%. Nodular BCC however has a complete response rate of 10–64%. Fluorescence microscopy studies suggest that the distribution of photosensitizer and depth of penetration of photosensitizer may be important factors in the poorer response of BCC and there is some evidence that BCCs less than 1 mm thick have a significantly higher cure rate than thicker tumours.

Squamous cell carcinoma

There have been few studies using PDT to treat SCC but there is a reported average CR rate of 72% using systemic porphyrin PDT and 0–67% using topical ALA PDT.

Radiotherapy

The use of radiotherapy for the treatment of precancer and skin cancer has declined over recent decades. This is mainly due to advances in dermatological and surgical techniques, particularly reconstructive surgery and Mohs' micrographic surgery. However, radiotherapy has an important role in the management of appropriately selected skin tumours.

The main advantages of radiotherapy are normal tissue preservation, particularly when treating tumours of the external ear, nose and periorbital regions; management of patients with tumour-positive surgical margins, perineural invasion and metastatic lymphadenopathy; and use without anaesthesia in those patients who are unfit for surgery.[7] Elderly patients are more favourable candi-

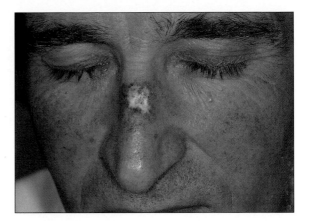

Figure 7.4
Hypopigmentation and atrophy years after radiotherapy.

dates for radiotherapy than younger patients because of the tendency for the generally good cosmetic outcome to decline over many years with the development of varying degrees of atrophy, hypopigmentation, telangiectasia and alopecia in the irradiated skin (Figure 7.4).

Early-stage skin cancer can be treated with orthovoltage radiotherapy, electron-beam radiation or interstitial therapy.[7] Orthovoltage radiotherapy has favourable beam characteristics for treating superficial tumours less than 5 mm thick, but orthovoltage units are slowly being phased out because of limited applications. At the same time high-energy linear accelerators, which can produce megavoltage photon and electron beams, are becoming more available. There are many different dose-fractionation protocols used but in general higher doses per fraction and fewer treatment sessions will cause more permanent normal tissue damage than using lower dosages per fraction over a longer time period. The convenience to the patient of fewer treatment sessions therefore needs to be balanced against cosmetic outcome. In addition skin cancers can be treated by inserting radioactive sources directly into the tumour – a technique called interstitial therapy or brachytherapy.

Tumours that recur following radiotherapy should be treated by other treatment modalities. Conversely, radiotherapy may be an effective treatment for tumours that recur after other treatment modalities. Patient selection is very important which is why collaboration between specialists and combined clinics involving dermatologists, plastic surgeons and radiation oncologists is a useful approach in the management of patients with difficult, complicated or high-risk skin cancers.

Bowen's disease

Complete reponse rates of 89–97% have been reported using radiotherapy to treat BD with good to excellent cosmetic results. Cox and Dyson looked at the wound healing on the lower leg after radiotherapy or cryotherapy for BD.[8] Fifty-nine lesions of BD on the lower leg were treated by external beam radiotherapy resulting in a 20% rate of failure to heal but a 100% complete tumour response. A field size > 4 cm had a greater than 50% risk of failure to heal. Only 2% of the cryotherapy-treated lesions failed to heal, although 6% had local recurrence compared with none in the radiotherapy group. Both of the lesions that failed to heal were shown to have residual BD histologically.

In another study four patients with erythroplasia of Queyrat were treated with soft X-ray therapy with all cases showing a complete response at 6 months, but one case had a local recurrence 8 months after therapy. Grabstald and Kelly reported a 90% complete response rate with small, noninfiltrating or superficially infiltrating cancers of the glans or prepuce treated by radiation therapy.[9] However, 40%

developed urethral stricture and late skin telangiectasia was seen in all patients. Radiation may be best reserved for resistant lesions when further surgery cannot be considered.

Basal cell carcinoma

Radiotherapy is used to treat many types of BCC and careful selection of patients and lesions can produce very high cure rates. Two large reviews of published studies suggest overall 5-year cure rates for primary BCC of 91.3% and for recurrent BCC of 90.2%.[10]

The problems of late onset atrophy, hypopigmentation and telangiectasia make radiotherapy less favourable in younger patients. In addition late fibrosis may cause epiphora and ectropion following treatment of lower eyelid and inner canthal lesions. It has been suggested that BCCs recurring following radiotherapy may behave more aggressively, but this may simply indicate that these lesions were initially an aggressive, high-risk type.

Squamous cell carcinoma

Radiotherapy alone produces cure rates for SCC which are comparable to other non-Mohs' treatments. In particular treatment of SCC with surgery followed by adjuvant radiotherapy is more effective than radiotherapy alone.[11] Radiotherapy is of value treating the large, rapidly growing SCCs and in those where surgery is contraindicated.

Melanoma

Radiotherapy has been advocated for the treatment of lentigo maligna in elderly patients for whom surgery and reconstruction were contraindicated or too difficult. A review of the literature yielded an average recurrence rate of 6.7%.[12] As well as the cosmetic disadvantages of atrophy, hypopigmentation and telangiectasia, there is a lack of histological assessment of the whole lesion to exclude a focus of lentigo maligna melanoma.

Topical 5-fluorouracil

Topical 5-fluorouracil is a fluorinated pyrimidine that was introduced as a new class of tumour-inhibitory compound in 1957. The specific indication for topical 5-FU is solar keratoses, but it is also used to treat warts, keratoacanthomas, BD, extramammary Paget's and erythroplasia of Queyrat.

Solar keratoses

The effectiveness of 5-FU has been established over the last 30 years. In the traditional method 5-FU is applied twice daily for 2–4 weeks. Individual lesions may be treated but if there is a field defect with numerous lesions close together then a thin, even coating is applied to the entire surface – the 5-FU selectively removing the sun-damaged areas. It usually produces excellent cosmetic results efficiently and economically. The conventional daily treatment regime for solar keratoses produces a response rate of approximately 93%.

A brisk inflammatory response following the application of 5-FU can result in unsightly and uncomfortable erosions, but many feel that this is required to produce a satisfactory result. This reaction may lead to rejection of the treatment or poor compliance. Modifications to concentration and frequency of application

have therefore been tried. Another variation is a weekly pulse regime. 5-Fluorouracil is applied morning and night on 1 day a week (this is increased to 2 days per week if progress is not satisfactory). This regime produced 98% clearing of solar keratoses in 10 patients in an average of 6.7 weeks with local irritation limited to erythema.[13]

The descriptions above, of some published approaches for the application of 5-FU, are amongst numerous in routine clinical practice. It is important that the patient has clear instructions and the use of information sheets are recommended. There are instructions included in the product package but they may

Table 7.1
Patient information sheet.

EFUDIX   10–14 day method

Efudix cream should only be applied to the affected skin.
You may apply it with a cotton bud.

Please avoid contact with your eyes.

Apply the cream to the affected area and leave it on for 12 hours. Overnight is a convenient time. You may cover it with a dressing or plaster if needed.

After 12 hours wash the cream off carefully.

Repeat this process daily until the skin becomes a bit red and sore – usually between 10 and 14 days.

Do remember to keep your next hospital appointment.

Chesterfield Royal Hospital
Dermatology Department

---

not be the same as the ones that the physician prefers to follow. Table 7.1 gives an example of patient information.

Bowen's disease

Recurrences are not infrequent and may arise from extensions of the carcinoma in situ into hair follicles. Sturm treated 41 lesions of BD in 39 patients with topical 5-FU (1–3%) applied twice a day for 4–12 weeks. He reported three recurrences (8%), all of which were successfully retreated with 5-FU. Extended courses may be required. Welch et al used iontophoresis to improve penetration:[14] 26 patients with 26 lesions of BD were treated twice a week for 4 weeks; 3 months after treatment the entire site was excised and subjected to step sectioning. They reported a 96% cure rate (25/26). Iontophoresis has the potential to deliver 5-FU more efficiently down adnexal structures to the follicular epithelium. Stone and Burge used once weekly application for a minimum of 3 months and found this to be a useful conservative way of controlling the disease in the lower limbs of the elderly.[15]

Basal cell carcinoma

Treatment of BCC by 5-FU is restricted by the depth of penetration of the drug. Reported response rates for superficial BCCs treated by topical 5-FU are 80–87% with up to 18 months' follow-up. When preceded by light curettage recurrence rates are reduced.[16] 5-Fluorouracil may be useful for low-risk extra-facial lesions and multiple superficial BCC on the trunk and limbs. Thicker, invasive lesions with follicular involvement are unlikely to respond.

Intralesional interferon

Interferons (IFNs) are a family of naturally occurring glycoproteins with antiviral, anti-proliferative and immunomodulatory effects. There have been a number of reports over the last few years of successful treatment with systemic or intralesional IFNs of a number of cutaneous malignancies including T-cell lymphoma, melanoma, Kaposi's sarcoma and BCC.

Basal cell carcinoma

In 1986 Greenway et al first described eight patients with superficial or nodular BCC successfully treated with intralesional IFN alpha-2b. Further studies have demonstrated a 67–81% complete response rate for superficial or nodular BCCs treated in this way.[17] A typical protocol involves $1.5–3 \times 10^6$ IU of IFN, three times a week for 4–8 weeks.

The use of IFNs is an interesting approach to the treatment of skin cancer. Suggested mechanisms of action include inhibition of tumour growth, specific cytotoxicity and induction of antitumour cellular immunity. At the present time the use of intralesional interferon is very expensive and time consuming but this approach is of considerable research interest.

Laser vaporization

The carbon dioxide laser, developed in 1964, emits continuous wave far-infrared radiation at 10 600 nm which is absorbed specifically by tissue water. The defocused beam heats tissue rapidly, converting intra- and extracellular water into steam, leaving charred tissue. This happens so quickly that there is minimal transfer of thermal energy to adjacent tissues. The carbon dioxide laser seals small blood vessels and lymphatics resulting in a bloodless field. If the beam passes over the tissue at a constant speed it can vaporize precisely and reproducibly thin layers of tissue. Several passes may be required to vaporize a cutaneous lesion. It requires experience to judge the endpoint of treatment. Superpulsing of the beam has allowed higher peak powers and shorter pulse durations.

The recently developed Erbium:YAG pulsed laser emits infrared radiation at 2940 nm, which is strongly absorbed by water. The depth of thermal damage is < 50 μm and is not as practical for the removal of thick lesions. Laser vaporization of premalignant and malignant cutaneous tumours is not yet considered a standard therapy, except possibly for actinic cheilitis, and should be confined to carefully selected patients.

Solar keratoses

The scanning carbon dioxide laser has been used for extensive and diffuse actinic keratoses and carcinoma in situ, particularly of the face.[18] There is histological evidence of regeneration of normal epithelium. A good cosmetic result is obtained but there are few data on long-term follow-up. It is an effective treatment for actinic cheilitis where the mucosal epithelium can be selectively destroyed.

Bowen's disease

Laser vaporization's usefulness for BD may be limited because of extension of the carcinoma in-situ down hair follicles and indeed experience has confirmed that thick or keratotic lesions are less likely to be completely ablated. However in selected cases of BD in awkward sites, such as the finger, it appears to be an effective option.[19]

In three cases of erythoplasia of Queyrat all patients achieved a complete response, maintained at 14–36 months' follow-up, with excellent functional and cosmetic results.

Basal cell carcinoma

There is relatively little work on this application but superficial lesions have been the target in most studies.[19] Curettage with carbon dioxide laser vaporization may be useful for large or multiple superficial BCC. They can be completely ablated by three passes of the high-energy superpulsed CO_2 laser as confirmed by histological evaluation.

Melanoma

Carbon dioxide laser ablation of cutaneous melanoma metastases may be a useful palliative option in patients with extensive disease when local excision is not feasible.[20]

Cryosurgery

History

Over 100 years ago James Arnott treated cancer by freezing tissue to −10°C with salt and ice solutions. Cure of early skin cancers and palliative benefits for advanced lesions were reported in 1901. Liquid nitrogen (−196°C) was introduced into practice in 1950 and with better delivery systems it has become the most popular refrigerant.

Cryobiology

When cells are frozen, ice crystals form extracellularly and then intracellularly, and the cells shrink following osmotic changes. This effect is greatest when freezing occurs rapidly. Slow thawing increases the mechanical injury. As the tissue thaws, endothelial cell damage leads to leakage and oedema, intravascular platelet aggregation and thrombus formation in capillaries and venules. Although temperatures of −20°C lead to the death of some cells, colder temperatures around −50°C seem to be more effective and are recommended for tumours.

Cell types vary in their sensitivity to cold. Keratinocytes are quite hardy but fibroblasts and collagen fibres are more so. Their relative resistance to freezing is of great benefit when treating tumours aggressively as the architectural scaffold of the tissue is preserved preventing distortion on healing. Melanocytes are easily killed, hence the rapid development of hypopigmentation, but cryosurgery is not useful in the treatment of primary melanoma because histological specimens are required.

Cryogenic lesion and healing

As the tissue thaws after tumouricidal doses of liquid nitrogen there is oedema, a dusky discolouration and small haemorrhages are seen. A narrow bright red halo is seen at the periphery. Oedema increases and blistering may appear followed within a few days by well-defined necrosis. This eschar may take weeks to separate and is frequently followed by a further eschar. During this time there is often leakage which may be extensive and either blood stained or semipurulent. Healing begins beneath the eschar and is unusual in several respects. The preserved collagen fibres maintain normal anatomy. Contraction is

rarely seen so that distortion of free edges, for example, eyelids, is not a problem. Hypertrophic scarring is equally rare even in areas normally prone to their development.

Repetition of the freeze–thaw cycle increases the certainty of cell death. These observations have led to a more uniform approach to the treatment of skin cancer. The tumour is normally frozen as quickly as possible and maintained in this stage for about 30 s. Thawing is unaided and the second freeze–thaw cycle is then initiated.

Understanding the development and shape of the cryolesion is important when treating skin cancer. Work on animals and humans shows that the isotherms lie close together when freezing is rapid. This means that lethal temperatures are found near to the base of the iceball after rapid freezing. To depths of about 6 mm the contour of the cryolesion is rounded but below this it becomes more triangular. Of the common BCCs 90% are 3 mm or less in depth and certainly for these the experimental data support the concept that lethal temperatures can readily be achieved at this depth.

Cryosurgical equipment

Three types of system are used, namely sprays (Figure 7.5a), probes (Figure 7.5b) and cotton buds. The latter are used chiefly for benign and premalignant lesions. The freezing characteristics of each method are different so that treatment schedules vary.

Sprays are open systems but the effect can be increased by using neoprene cones to confine the nitrogen stream. This system is particularly suited to treating tumours on convex or irregular surfaces. Probes are applied to the skin with a lubricating jelly at the interface. The metal surface cools down as the cryogen passes through the probe to be

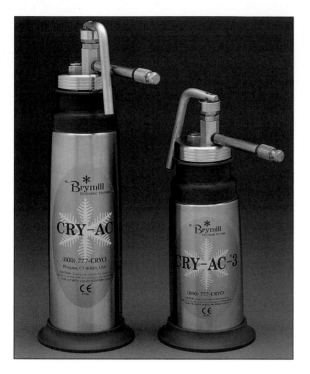

Figure 7.5a
A modern liquid nitrogen cryospray.

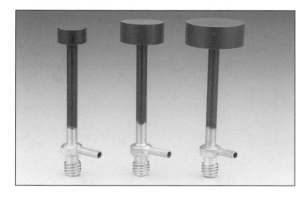

Figure 7.5b
Liquid nitrogen cryoprobes.

vented downstream. Pressure can be applied on the probe increasing the freezing effect. Cotton buds are dipped into a flask of the liquid and pressed onto the lesion. Variables include the tightness of the cotton and how firmly the bud is pressed on the lesion.

Monitoring and treatment techniques

Cryosurgeons use experience and knowledge of the tumour characteristics to plan an appropriate strategy. The stages of freezing can be judged by palpation; in some sites this is assisted by fixation of the tissues to bone. Depth is also gauged by the relationship to the lateral spread of freeze from the edge of the probe or neoprene cone.

Some practitioners monitor temperature changes by inserting a needle under the tumour to act as a thermocouple or measure of tissue electrical resistance. In the latter case this increases abruptly at a point when extracellular water crystallizes. One problem here is the difficulty of knowing whether the needle is exactly beneath the tumour.

The standard approach for tumours up to about 1.5 cm is to mark the tumour border in ink and then to draw a further line 4–5 mm from the clinical margin. An open spray is then applied to the centre of the tumour continuously until the ice margin spreads to the outer ink line. The ice ball is then maintained for 30 s by intermittent spraying. Thawing for several minutes is followed by a repeat of the same cycle. If a cone is used it should be chosen to have a diameter equal to that of the tumour. The usual second cycle is given after thawing. Some experts mould adhesive putty to circumscribe the lesion with a suitable margin and apply the nitrogen within those confines.

The probe technique requires the choice of a probe the same size as the tumour, cooling it for a few minutes and then applying it firmly with lubricating jelly to the tumour surface.

The ice front gradually extends to the predetermined treatment margin. The length of freeze depends on the tumour type, monitoring information, palpation and so on.

Side-effects

Swelling is worst in areas of lax tissue. It is common for the eye to close with oedema when tumours are treated in this vicinity and the lip may become hugely swollen (Figure 7.6). Oozing often accompanies the oedema and repeated dressing changes are required. Delayed bleeding is very rare but may occur at 14 days. It usually involves an artery and may be profuse requiring urgent attention.

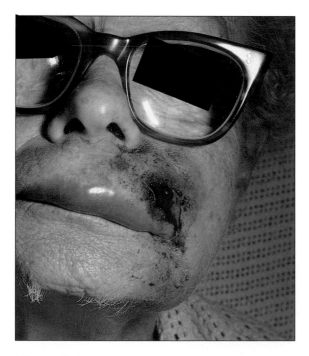

Figure 7.6
Swelling of the lip 24 h after tumour doses of cryotherapy.

Some pain is experienced at the onset of freezing but a more severe pain may occur after thawing lasting minutes to hours. The ear, lips, temple and scalp are particularly sensitive. Damage to other skin structures may lead to loss of sweat and sebaceous glands and alopecia. The texture of the skin compares favourably with surgical scars and hypertrophy is rare and temporary.

Cartilage is relatively resistant to damage and the shape of the helix or nasal cartilage is preserved but aggressive freezing may produce notching: if the tumour has already invaded cartilage it will be shed as part of the inflammatory response. Deep freezing over bone may lead to necrosis and over tendons has caused rupture. This is particularly relevant for the small tendons on the dorsum of the fingers. Care is needed around the proximal nailfold to avoid damage to the matrix with permanent nail dystrophy. In common with most destructive therapies healing on the lower leg may be very slow.

Patient selection

Certain patients are particularly suited to this form of treatment:

- all ages – even patients in poor health or at home,
- Caucasians – hyper- and hypopigmentation are less in this group,
- those on anticoagulants,
- individuals allergic to local anaesthesia,
- patients who are high-risk because of blood-borne infections.

There are contra-indications for patients with concomitant diseases such as cold urticaria, cryoglobulinaemia, pyoderma gangrenosum and Raynaud's disease.

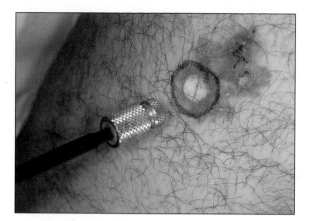

Figure 7.7
Treating Bowen's disease with overlapping
circles of cryosurgery.

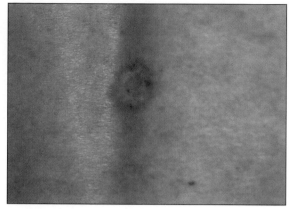

Figure 7.8
Six months after cryosurgery to a superficial
basal cell carcinoma on the back.

Solar keratosis

Cryosurgery is one of the best options with
response rates of 98% using either the spray or
cotton bud method applying the nitrogen for
5–10 s. Multiple lesions can be treated. Hyperkeratotic lesions will normally be treated
with other modalities. Actinic cheilitis is also
responsive in the early stages.

Bowen's disease

This method is not superior to curettage or
5-FU with regard to persistence of disease
around follicles but when freezes of up to 30 s
are used the recurrence rate at 1 year is about
10%. The lesions of BD can be treated with
sprays, probes or even cotton buds dipped into
liquid nitrogen. The margin of normal skin
treated is much smaller than for malignant
disease and 1–2 mm is usually sufficient. For
larger lesions the use of overlapping treatment
circles can be considered (Figure 7.7).

Basal cell carcinoma

In experienced hands and for selected tumours
cryosurgery gives good cure rates (Figure 7.8).
Certain factors make malignancies particularly suitable for this treatment:

- well-defined tumours up to 1.5 cm,
- superficial truncal type BCC even if bigger
  than 1.5 cm,
- tumours on sites with poor skin mobility
  or sites prone to keloid,
- tumours recurring following radiotherapy,
- multiple tumours, for example, Gorlin's
  syndrome or postirradiation to the back,
- some tumours of the ear, eyelid or nose
  where surgery may produce mutilation.

Conversely there are some tumours which
are less suitable for this type of treatment:

- tumours greater than 1.5 cm,
- tumours recurrent after cryosurgery,
- tumours with a high recurrence rate, for

example, nasolabial fold, pre-auricular area,

- some histological types, particularly morphoeic BCC.

Cure rates

Comparison between studies is hampered by different lesions and site selection. Indeed some studies do not separate BCC from SCC. Overall cryosurgery is a safe and effective method for dealing with skin cancer giving good cosmetic results and an overall cure rate of 95–99% in the majority of studies.[21] Some studies use shave or curettage followed by freezing while others use double freeze–thaw cycles with or without the debulking procedure. Clinical experience determines which method to use and care must be taken not to overtreat (for example, thin BCCs on the back) nor to undertreat (for example, deep tumours of the nasolabial fold). Some studies such as that of Zacarian in the USA looked at very large numbers and found 97.3% cure rate in 4228 tumours.

Holt in the UK found 97% cure in 279 skin cancers over 5 years.[22] Graham had a 98.2% cure rate in 3593 new tumours. In some literature there are lower cure rates on the scalp, nasolabial fold, lips and eyelid and this may reflect inadequate freezing. This is borne out by a detailed study on BCC of the eyelid, in which 222 well-defined tumours were treated aggressively; none recurred and half the patients were followed up for over 5 years.[23]

Large tumours (2 cm or more) have a slightly lower cure rate and this is so for all modalities of treatment. A recent paper which used aggressive cryosurgery for large tumours on the nose emphasized how good this treatment is even in this difficult clinical situation.[24] Recurrent tumours are always more difficult

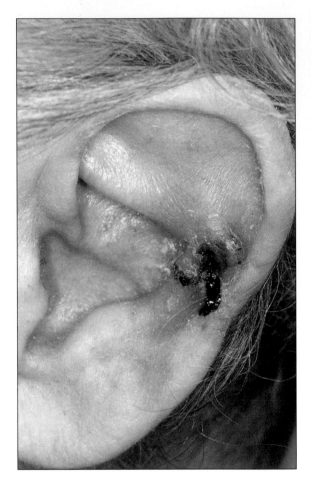

Figure 7.9
Squamous cell carcinoma before cryotherapy.

to treat and cryosurgery is not generally recommended. However when aggressive freezing was used a cure rate of 88% was achieved in 164 cases treated over a 16-year period.

Squamous cell carcinoma

Patient selection is exactly the same as for BCC. The same caveats apply and as the treat-

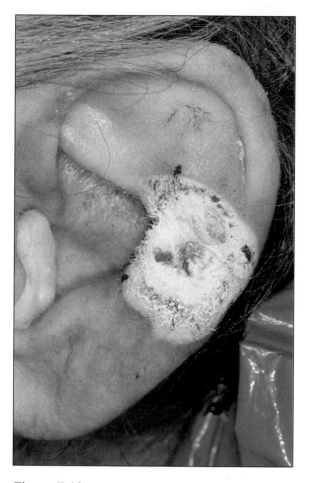

Figure 7.10
Same lesion as shown in Figure 7.9 immediately after freezing.

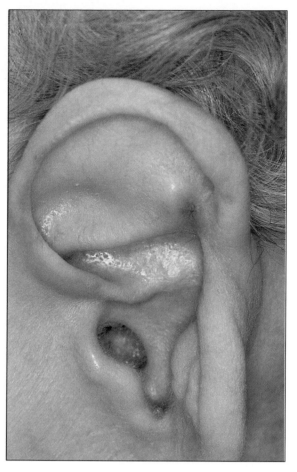

Figure 7.11
Same lesion as shown in Figure 7.9 4 months after treatment.

ment schedules are similar one can anticipate the same profile of side-effects. Figures 7.9–7.11 show successful treatment of an SCC of the ear in a 90-year-old patient in a nursing home where other forms of treatment were less appropriate. Lesion selection is perhaps more difficult than for BCC. These tumours are intrinsically more worrying. The earliest SCCs which derive from solar keratosis can be treated with a relatively nonaggressive approach. However larger and less well-differentiated tumours demand an aggressive treatment. Surgical excision or radiotherapy will normally be best but if conditions are right, cryosurgery it can be used to good effect. Whereas small, well-differentiated lesions on the scalp or back of the hand may be suitable, those on the lip and ear are unlikely to be so.

Patient information and wound care

It is usual to issue an information leaflet as the degree of swelling comes as a surprise. The leaflet should describe the after-effects and give a contact telephone number to ring if there is undue concern. It should always outline wound care. Daily washing with saline or tap water and gauze pads to absorb exudate are the mainstay of treatment.

References

1. Graham JH, Helwig EB (1973) Erythroplasia of Queyrat. A clinico-pathologic and histochemical study, *Cancer* **32**:1396–1414.
2. Rowe DE, Carroll RJ, Day CL Jr (1989) Long-term recurrence rates in previously untreated (primary) basal cell carcinoma: implications for patient follow-up, *J Dermatol Surg Oncol* **15**:315–28.
3. Freeman RG, Knox JM, Heaton CL (1964) A statistical study of 1341 skin tumours comparing results obtained with irradiation, surgery and curettage followed by electrodesiccation. The treatment of skin cancer, *Cancer* **17**:535–8.
4. Stables GI (in press) Photodynamic therapy, *J Dermatol Treat*.
5. Morton CA, Whitehurst C, Moseley H et al (1996) Comparison of photodynamic therapy with cryotherapy in the treatment of Bowen's disease, *Br J Dermatol* **135**:766–71.
6. Stables GI, Stringer MR, Robinson DJ et al (1997) Large patches of Bowen's disease treated by topical aminolaevulinic acid photodynamic therapy, *Br J Dermatol* **136**:957–60.
7. Morrison WH, Garden AS, Ang KK (1997) Radiation therapy for nonmelanoma skin carcinomas, *Clin Plast Surg* **24**:719–29.
8. Cox NH, Dyson P (1995) Wound healing on the lower leg after radiotherapy or cryotherapy of Bowen's disease and other malignant skin lesions, *Br J Dermatol* **133**:60–5.
9. Grabstald H, Kelley CD (1980) Radiation therapy of penile cancer, *Urology* **15**:575–6.
10. Rowe DE, Carroll RJ, Day CL Jr (1989) Long-term recurrence rates in previously untreated (primary) basal cell carcinoma: implications for patient follow-up, *J Dermatol Surg Oncol* **15**:315–28.
11. Shimm DS, Wilder RB (1991) Radiation therapy for squamous cell carcinoma of the skin, *Am J Clin Oncol* **14**:383–6.
12. Gaspar ZS, Dawber RP (1997) Treatment of lentigo maligna, *Australas J Dermatol* **38**:1–6.
13. Pearlman DL (1991) Weekly pulse dosing: effective and comfortable topical 5-fluorouracil treatment of multiple facial actinic keratoses, *J Am Acad Dermatol* **25**:665–7.
14. Welch ML, Grabski WJ, McCollough ML et al (1997) 5-Fluorouracil iontophoretic therapy for Bowen's disease, *J Am Acad Dermatol* **36**:956–8.
15. Stone N, Burge S (1999) Bowen's disease of the leg treated by weekly pulses of 5-fluorouracil cream, *Br J Dermatol* **140**:987–8.
16. Epstein E (1985) Fluorouracil paste treatment of thin basal cell carcinomas, *Arch Dermatol* **121**:207–13.
17. Chimenti S, Peris K, Di Cristofaro S et al (1995) Use of recombinant interferon alfa-2b in the treatment of basal cell carcinoma, *Dermatology* **190**:214–17.
18. Trimas SJ, Ellis DA, Metz RD (1997) The carbon dioxide laser. An alternative for the treatment of actinically damaged skin, *Dermatol Surg* **23**:885–9.
19. Humphreys TR, Malhotra R, Scharf MJ et al (1998) Treatment of superficial basal cell carcinoma and squamous cell carcinoma in-situ with a high-energy pulsed carbon dioxide laser, *Arch Dermatol* **134**:1247–52.
20. Strobbe LJ, Nieweg OE, Kroon BB (1997) Carbon dioxide laser for cutaneous melanoma

metastases: indications and limitations, *Eur J Surg Oncol* **23**:435–8.

21. McIntosh G, Osbourne D (1983) Basal cell carcinoma: a review of treatment results with special reference to cryosurgery, *Postgrad Med J* **59**:698–701.

22. Holt PSA (1988) Cryotherapy for skin cancer. Results over a five year period using liquid nitrogen spray, *Br J Dermatol* **119**:231–40.

23. Lindgren G, Larko O (1997) Long term follow-up of cryosurgery of basal cell carcinoma of the eyelid, *JAAD* **36**:742–6.

24. Nordin P, Larko O, Stenquist B (1997) Five year results of curettage cryosurgery of selected large primary basal cell carcinomas of the nose: An alternative treatment in a geographical area unserved by Mohs' surgery, *Br J Dermatol* **136**:180–3.

Bibliography

Kuflik EG, Gage AA (eds) (1990) *Cryosurgical Treatment for Skin Cancer* (Igaku Shoin).

8 Treatment 2 – excisional surgery

Introduction

Excisional surgery with a scalpel remains the most commonly performed procedure for specialists who are involved with the treatment of skin cancer. The indications have been discussed in earlier chapters along with its advantages and limitations. Good cosmetic results and effective tumour removal must be achieved and here the essentials of good technique are discussed.

Excisional surgery

Blade to skin

Each incision should be made as a single continuous sweep rather than a series of small nicks. The incision lines should meet neatly without crossing at the tip and this is done by starting and finishing each sweep with the blade held vertically. It is also important to hold the blade at 90° to the skin, not angled inwards. This will produce a defect with vertical sides that is easier to close because there is no residual dermis or fat in the way.

Lines of excision

Plan the incision with the patient seated in a relaxed posture and mark important cosmetic boundaries, skin creases and incision lines before giving the anaesthetic, because the injection will produce oedema and temporary paralysis of facial expression muscles and hence obscure these lines. Remember to anaesthetize both the lesion and surrounding skin so the area can be undermined if necessary. Draw on the skin using a purpose-made marker pen or Bonney's blue ink (a mixture of gentian violet and malachite green) and avoid other ink pigments because these may become tattooed into the skin.

Good scar cosmesis

A good scar is smooth, flat, narrow and as short as possible. Scars are never as strong as the surrounding normal skin and at the time of suture removal the wound has only 5% of its unwounded strength. The risk of a scar stretching or a wound falling apart can be reduced by providing additional support in the form of subcutaneous sutures during closure and using tape strips after surface suture removal. Stretching is minimized by placing the wound parallel to the wrinkle or crease lines. These lines run parallel to the dermal collagen bundles and perpendicular to the direction of contraction of the underlying muscles. On the limbs most experts recommend that the wound direction should follow skin crease lines but some prefer to make the incision run in the direction of the long axis of the limb.

Choice of excision margins

When treating patients with skin cancer, it is imperative not to compromise the adequacy of the excision to make the repair easier. A margin of apparently uninvolved skin must be removed with the tumour to guard against the possibility of the tumour extending beyond the visible margin. When looking for the tumour margin the patient should be examined in a good light, with magnification if necessary. The size of this margin has been discussed in Chapters 3–5. The role of microscopically controlled excision of basal cell carcinomas (BCCs) (Mohs' surgery) is discussed below. The need to remove a margin of normal skin means that excision of even a small tumour will result in a significant defect. For example, removal of an 8 mm diameter BCC with a 4 mm margin will produce a 16 mm diameter defect.

Depth of excision

Obviously the depth of excision should be below that of the tumour. Most BCCs do not spread beyond the dermis so that excision of the skin down to fat (that is, subcutaneous tissue) is normally all that is required. This means cutting through the full thickness of the dermis. On the back this is 5–8 mm thick whereas on the face the dermis is only 1–4 mm thick. Excisions down to fat will rarely result in exposure or potential damage to important structures unless the subject is extremely thin. Excision down to deep fascia is relatively easy to do in thin individuals and will result in exposure of named nerves and arteries at some sites and thus a knowledge of the superficial anatomy is essential.

Undermining

Once the tumour has been excised the defect can be closed. At most sites it will be necessary to pull the skin edges together, resulting in some tension. Skin mobility at the wound edge can be increased by undermining or separating the full thickness of skin (that is, the epidermis, dermis and superficial fat) from the underlying tissues. This process of undermining the skin to increase mobility has to be done at different levels depending on the body site (Table 8.1).

Undermining must be done under full vision to avoid damaging large vessels or nerves. The best technique is to tunnel into the fat with round-ended scissors separating the strands of fatty tissue by repeatedly opening the scissors. Sometimes it is possible to form an adjacent tunnel and the wall between the two tunnels trimmed carefully with scissors if necessary. When possible leave small vessels connecting the deeper tissues and skin intact as these deliver blood to the skin from the deep dermal plexus. On the trunk and limbs it is usually easiest to undermine in the deep fat. Undermining just above the deep fascia may involve

Table 8.1
Undermining levels.

Site	Undermining level
Face	Mid fat
Nose	Beneath muscles of facial expression and above the periosteum/perichondrium
Scalp	Subgaleal plane
Forehead	Beneath the deep frontalis fascia
Trunk and limbs	Deep fat or just above deep fascia

operating down a deep hole in some individuals and is painful unless the fascia is also anaesthetized.

On the scalp undermine beneath the galea. This well-defined fibrous sheath is the extension of the two layers of fascia that envelop the frontalis muscle on the forehead and the occipital muscle posteriorly. Above the galea lie fat, hair follicles and blood vessels; beneath the galea are the periosteum and bony skull. Between the galea and the underlying periosteum is the subgaleal plane, a largely blood-vessel-free potential space. The only structures that may be found at this site are emissary veins connecting the intracranial venous sinuses and scalp veins. These vary in size and position in different individuals; a common one is the parietal emissary vein which crosses the subgaleal space at the back of the scalp Undermining increases local tissue injury in the short term and patients may experience more bruising and swelling as a result. Warn them of the possible consequences of surgery.

Reconstruction

A defect created by excision of a tumour can be managed in several ways. A general rule is to keep the method as simple as possible and primary closure is ideal so long as it does not produce undue tension or distortion. The method chosen is frequently determined by the site and size of the defect. At sites such as the medial canthus, temple, nasolabial fold and antehelix second-intention healing can be used if the patient wishes to avoid a further procedure and accepts the need for repeat dressings. If the wound is small enough direct closure is usually possible at all sites. Flaps can be used to preserve landmarks, minimize scar length and facilitate closure when this is not possible

by direct closure. Grafts are used if there is no tissue movement and flap repair is therefore impossible. In comparison with flaps, grafts are technically easier to perform but generally produce inferior cosmetic results because they do not use adjacent matching skin to cover the defect.

Primary closure

All wounds, except the smallest should be sutured in layers. Deep absorbable sutures are inserted to bring the skin edges into apposition and then superficial sutures of monofilament material are placed with just sufficient tension to hold the skin edges together and prevent unnecessary movement. These superficial sutures can be removed after only a few days as the deep sutures remain in situ to maintain the strength needed for wound healing.

Oval excisions and dog-ear repair

Rather than assume that all lesions should be removed by elliptical excision it is frequently better to excise tumours with only the necessary margin of normal skin as a circle. After tumour removal the shape of the excised area is remodelled by the surrounding skin turgor resulting in a circular or oval defect, the long axis of which lies parallel to the natural skin tension lines. The area around the wound can then be undermined and the optimal direction or method of closure assessed using two skin hooks to manipulate the wound edges. When there is sufficient mobility to allow the skin edges to be brought together without excessive tension and without distorting free skin margins such as the lid or lip, deep sutures should be placed centrally. Closure of the circular wound will leave dog ears or mounds

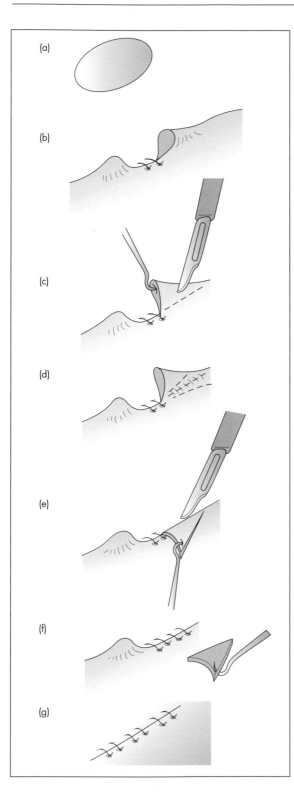

Figure 8.1
Dog-ear repair. The oval or circular shaped wound (a) is closed with interrupted subcutaneous and surface sutures as required in the appropriate direction so that the scar will follow the skin creases (b). The resulting repair has a mound of redundant skin at either end – the dog ears. Gentle traction on the dog ear using a skin hook identifies where the incision should be made to join the wound edge with the natural apex of the dog ear (c). This line is scored with a scalpel (d) and the full thickness of skin cut with scalpel or scissors. The piece of redundant skin is then draped over the wound edge (e) and the second incision made to complete the removal of the redundant triangle of skin (f). The other end of the wound is treated in the same way (g). (Reproduced with permission from Lawrence C (1996) *An Introduction to Dermatological Surgery* (Blackwell Science: Oxford).)

of skin at the ends of the wound which can be removed as necessary (Figure 8.1). The direction of the dog ear can be designed by the operator so that the scar will run in an adjacent skin crease or cosmetic boundary and is determined by the first incision (Figure 8.2). The length of the repair is determined by the amount of tissue that needs to be removed to ensure that the wound lies flat. The technique can be adapted to avoid cutting into an important adjacent structure such as the eye or nose by creating two dog ears angled at approximately 60° away from the critical structure. This is usually referred to as a W or M plasty.

Special sites

Lip

If the defect is close to the lip, mark the vermilion border before local anaesthetic injection in case this needs to be incised. It is essential when suturing the lip edge that the match is perfect because a stepped vermilion border looks strange and is difficult to disguise. Skin marker may come off during the procedure, therefore, mark the vermilion edge adjacent to the excision using a fine suture whilst the skin marker is visible and the skin is numb. Alternatively tattoo the vermilion edge using methylene blue and this will be completely absorbed after 7–14 days. Elliptical excisions around the lips should be placed in the radial perioral wrinkle lines to avoid unacceptable elevation of the vermilion border.

Lower leg

Wounds on the lower leg heal relatively slowly and healing is frequently delayed by coexisting venous oedema and arterial insufficiency. In general flaps are much less likely to survive on the leg and should be avoided at this site. The tight skin may prevent direct closure and techniques to increase skin mobility such as multiple relaxing incisions should be considered. Alternatively skin grafts (see below) may be required to cover larger defects.

Around the eyes

Excisions above the eyebrow may result in pronounced eyebrow lift producing a quizzical appearance. Whilst this normally disappears with time it should be avoided by using measures such as a flap repair from the temple or by adjusting the direction of closure so that the defect is closed with the long axis running parallel to the radial peri-orbital crease lines. On the lower eyelid the excision should not follow the skin creases if this risks everting the lower eyelid. A vertically orientated scar is better. This is a particular hazard in older people with poor eyelid tension.

Skin grafts

Full thickness grafts

A full thickness rather than a split skin graft is used when a superior cosmetic result and greater repair strength are important (Figure 8.3). Donor skin can be taken from any site with spare matching skin[1] although the skin from behind and in front of the ear, nasolabial fold, upper eyelid, inner aspect of the upper arm, lower abdominal wall and supraclavicular fossa is most frequently used. Ideally the donor skin should have similar dermal thickness, surface markings and weathering characteristics as the recipient site. A template of the defect site is made and this is used to mark out the area of the donor skin that needs to be removed. The donor skin is excised down to fat and the fat remaining on the under surface of the graft is trimmed off to prevent this hindering new blood vessel penetration. Edge sutures prevent shearing forces dislodging the graft, and a pressure dressing held in place using tie-over sutures is used to prevent a haematoma lifting the graft off the recipient site. Tie-over sutures are not used by all surgeons and for small grafts some other method of applying pressure may be used. There is no theoretical limitation to the size of a full thickness graft; graft size depends on how much donor skin can be harvested. Grafts take best on dermis and granulation tissue. They will just survive on fat, perichondrium and periosteum, but will perish on exposed bone, tendon, joint capsule

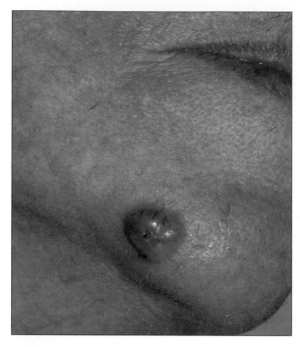

(a)

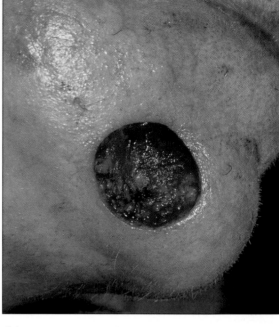

(b)

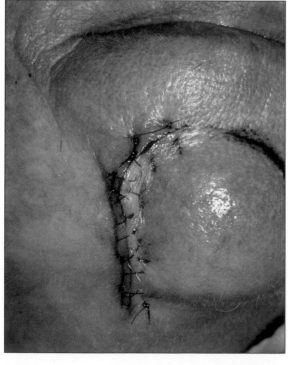

(c)

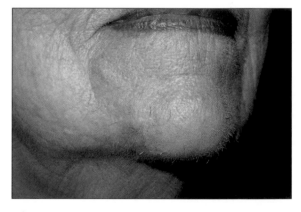

(d)

Figure 8.2
Tumour excision with dog-ear repair. This
basal cell carcinoma on the side of the
chin (a) was excised and the circular defect
remaining (b) closed so that the closure line
ran in the direction of the mentolabial
crease (c). In this way the final scar was
relatively invisible (d).

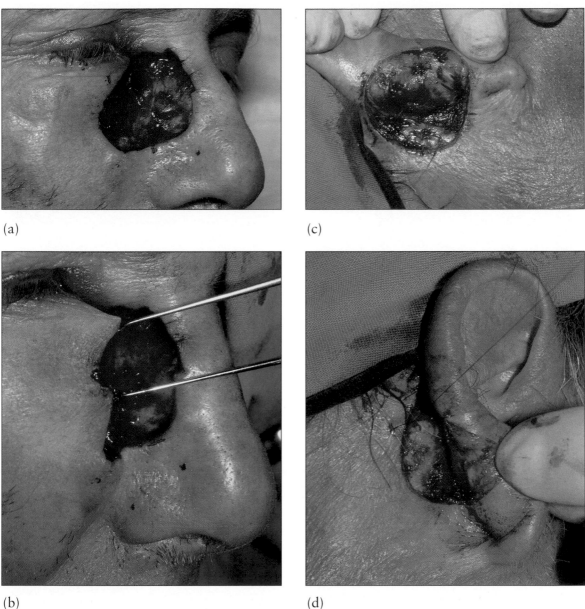

(a)

(c)

(b)

(d)

Figure 8.3
Full thickness graft. This defect on the side of the nose remained after basal cell carcinoma
excision (a). There was not enough loose skin for it to be closed by advancing the cheek (b). A
full thickness graft was therefore taken from behind the ear (c). The defect was covered by
suturing the edges together and thereby pinning the ear further back on to the scalp (d) but not
producing a noticeable scar.

continued

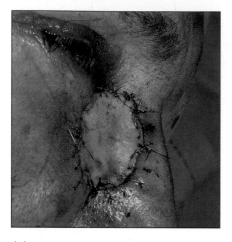

(e)

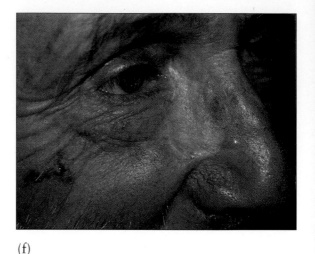

(f)

Figure 8.3 *continued*
Full thickness graft. The graft was sutured into place (e). The result was satisfactory 2 years later (f) but the grafted skin always looks different from the surrounding skin.

or cartilage. At some sites, for example, tip of nose, full thickness grafts are too thin and leave a depressed and rather unsatisfactory cosmetic result. It may be possible to allow granulation for a week prior to grafting. Alternatively, composite grafts containing skin and perichondrium, are better at this site as they contract less, induce new cartilage formation and maintain their thickness and epidermal appendages,[2] more readily than full thickness grafts.

Split skin grafts

A split graft involves slicing off a 0.2–0.45 mm thick layer of skin through the dermis, using a hand-held Humby knife or a mechanical dermatome, leaving behind the lower half of the adnexal and follicular structures. Epidermal cells then migrate from these adnexal structures to re-epithelialize the donor site. Split skin graft size is not usually limited by the availability of skin and thus they may be used to cover very large wounds. Split skin is also slightly transparent. This means that it can be used to cover tumour excision sites, where the adequacy of excision is dubious, so that a recurrence can be identified sooner than after a full thickness graft or flap closure. The disadvantages of split skin grafts are pain, poor healing of the donor site, the relatively poor cosmetic result and greater graft shrinkage. Meshing, or cutting multiple parallel slits in the graft, allows it to expand when stretched, rather like a fishnet stocking (Figure 8.4). The gaps fill up with epithelium that has migrated from the surrounding graft. A meshed graft will therefore cover a wider area than a similar sized unmeshed graft, conform to cover an uneven contour (for example, ear) and more importantly, especially on the lower leg, permit exudate to drain through the gaps. The common donor sites for split skin grafts include the upper arm, upper thigh and

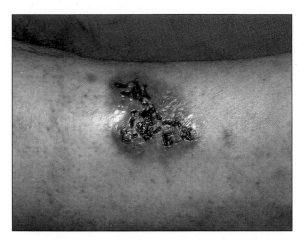

(a)

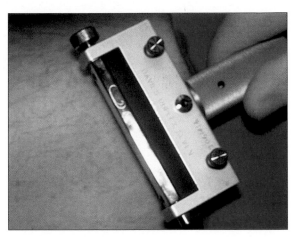

(b)

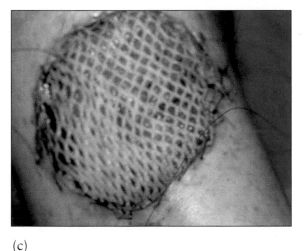

(c)

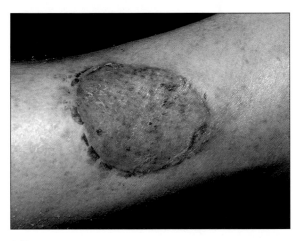

(d)

Figure 8.4
Meshed split skin graft. This patch of Bowen's disease (a) was excised and a split skin graft harvested using a power dermatome from the thigh skin (b). The skin was meshed and placed on the defect (c); (d) shows the appearance 1 month later.

abdominal wall. The donor site can be anaesthetized painlessly and effectively using EMLA cream and heals faster and painlessly when a calcium alginate or semi-permeable adhesive polyurethane film dressing is used.

Complications of grafts

Grafts fail because of infection or poor blood supply. Infection can be minimized by checking bacteriology pre-operatively and treating any pathogens present before attempting surgery. Pathogens are particularly likely to be present if the tumour surface is ulcerated or crusted. The use of prophylactic antibiotics after surgery to prevent wound infections is not required. In the first 3 days grafts receive their nutrients by diffusion. After 3 days blood vessels grow into the graft from the base and side of the wound. The development of haematoma or seroma under the graft will therefore act as barrier to new blood vessel penetration. Graft necrosis due to ischaemia occurs because of faulty technique, that is, incorrect homeostasis, suturing or wound care, or because the recipient site has a poor blood supply, for example, on the lower leg, or at radiotherapy treated sites. Smokers are at greater risk because cigarette smoking reduces cutaneous blood supply and should be avoided 2 days before and 7 days after surgery. All grafts contract and this may lead to ectropion on the lower eyelid. Grafts at critical sites are normally made 10–25% bigger than the defect in anticipation of this event. Depressed graft scars can sometimes be elevated by the injection of autograft fat under the graft.[3]

Flaps

Types

A flap is a piece of skin of full thickness which is moved to cover a nearby defect whilst receiving its blood supply from its origin via a pedicle. The vast majority of skin flaps used by dermatologists obtain their blood supply from the reticular dermal blood supply inherent in the skin pedicle, or in the case of island pedicle flaps (Figure 8.5) from the perforating vessels in the subdermal plexus. Flaps based on the inherent dermal vessels must therefore have a broad pedicle with a length-to-width ratio usually not exceeding 3:1. These flaps are categorized as advancement, rotation or transposition in type according to how the flap is moved to cover the defect. By contrast axial pattern flaps are designed to obtain their blood supply from one named artery and are rarely used by dermatologists, with the possible exception of the midline forehead flap which is based on the supratrochlear artery.

As the flap is moved to close the defect, a secondary defect is created which also has to be covered. The trick is to design the flap so that this secondary defect occurs where there is enough spare skin to allow the secondary defect to be closed. Thus, on the face most flaps will exploit any redundant skin present on the glabella, nasolabial fold, front of the ear, neck and cheek.

Uses

Advancement flaps (Figure 8.6) are simple to conceive but have limited use because the flaps have limited mobility. In some instances the defect is only covered by stretching the flap rather than transferring the tension to an area of lax skin. Rotation flaps usually require both advancement and rotation about a pivotal point on a broad pedicle. Mobility is frequently limited and long incisions and extensive undermining may be required to mobilize sufficient tissue; the secondary defect is closed last. Transposition flaps provide the greatest mobility and are different from the other two types because the secondary defect is closed first. As a result the flap is pushed rather than dragged into the defect. Thus, in a properly designed transposition flap virtually all the tension can be placed on the secondary defect rather than the flap. Different techniques can be used for many repairs although some techniques[4] are inherently suited to the nose (Figure 8.7), chin, eyelid, ear, forehead, scalp, cheeks and lip.

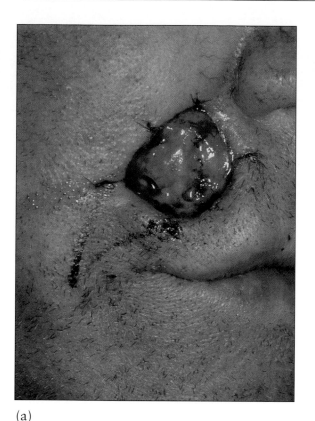

(a)

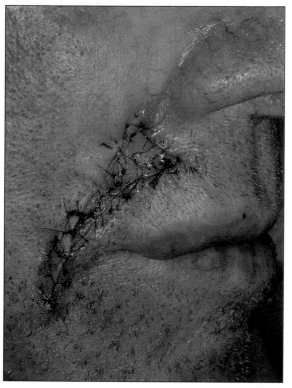

(b)

Figure 8.5
Island pedicle flap. This defect on the upper lip (a) remained after basal cell carcinoma
excision. Because it is very easy to produce a scar that distorts the upper lip if the defect is
closed directly this defect has to be closed by pulling up the loose skin at the side of the lip.
Using a flap which is not connected to the surrounding skin but gets its blood supply from the
underlying dermal pedicle a piece of skin can be moved into position without distorting the lip
margin (b).

Complications of flaps

Ischaemic necrosis of the flap (Figure 8.8)
usually occurs because of excessive tension
resulting from poor design or mobility.
Secondary infection is also more common if
the flap has a poor blood supply. On the head
and neck blood supply is excellent at all sites
but on the trunk and lower limb flap repair
fails because of the relatively poor blood
supply. Cigarette smokers are more vulnerable
to flap or graft necrosis than nonsmokers. This
risk can be minimized if smokers significantly
reduce cigarette consumption 2 days before
and 7 days after surgery. An obtrusive scar
line, particularly on the nose, can be improved
by dermabrasion or scalpel sculpturing 6
weeks after surgery.

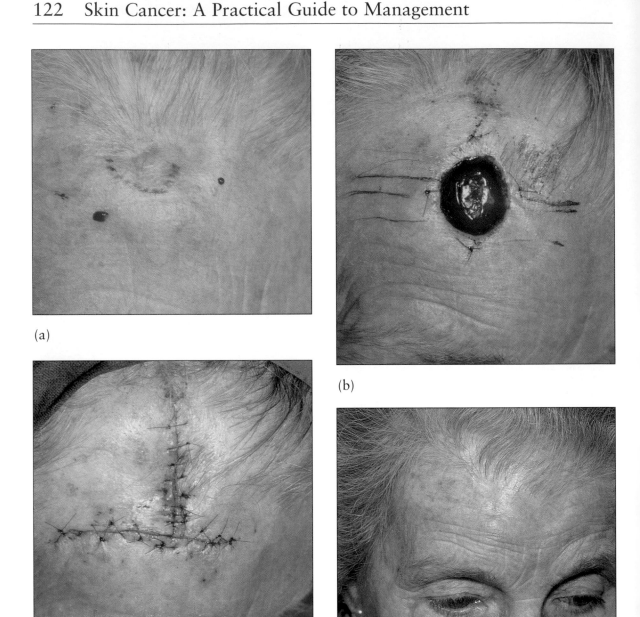

(a)

(b)

(c)

(d)

Figure 8.6
O–T flap repair of a forehead defect. This basal cell carcinoma on the forehead (a) was excised
(b) and the defect closed by advancing skin from either side (c). Rather than extend the closure
line down onto the forehead it was possible to adapt the closure so that only the skin above
the defect was moved. This is called an O–T repair and is useful when closing defects adjacent
to important structures such as the lip, eyelid or nose. The resulting scar was largely hidden in
the scalp (d).

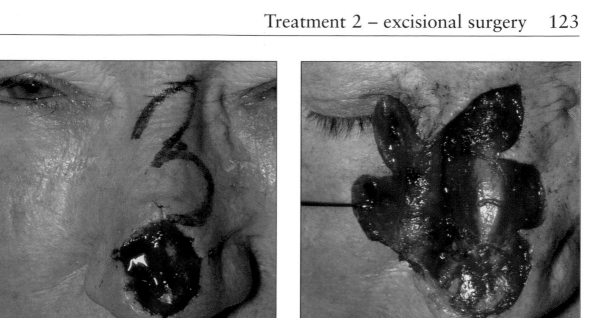

(a)   (b)

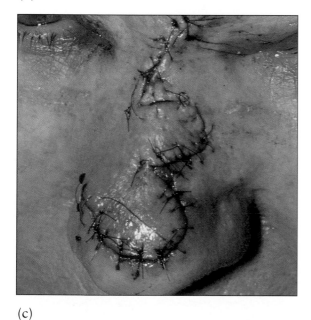

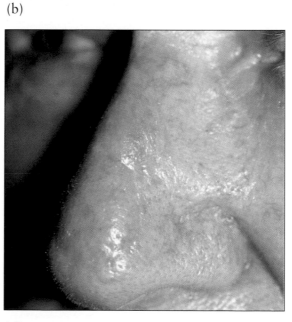

(c)   (d)

Figure 8.7
Bilobed flap on the nose. This defect near the tip of the nose (a) was covered using a bilobed flap designed to cover the defect by exploiting the looser skin higher up on the side of the nose. Both parts of the flap were raised together (b), transposed in the defect and the secondary defect and the tertiary defect were closed directly (c). The cosmetic result at 6 months was good (d).

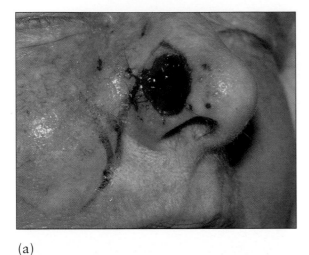

(a)

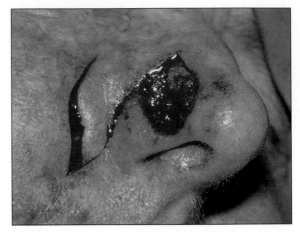

(b)

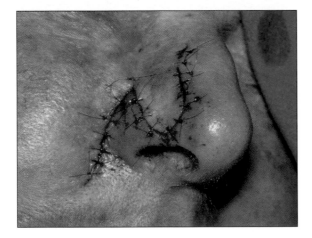

(c)

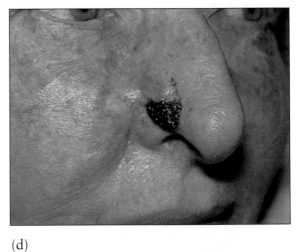

(d)

Figure 8.8
Complications – tip necrosis of a nasolabial
transposition flap. This defect on the side of
the nose (a) was closed using a type of
transposition flap called a nasolabial flap
that uses the spare skin on the cheek next to
the nasolabial fold (b). The flap looked fine
when finished (c) but the tip had necrosed at
suture removal (d). Fortunately the cosmetic
result was still satisfactory after the area was
allowed to heal by secondary intention (e).

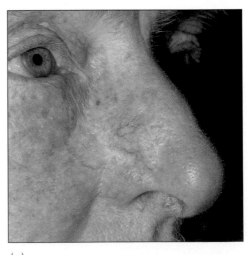

(e)

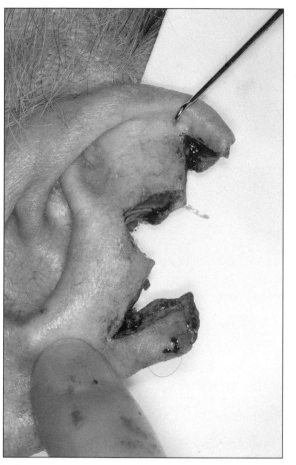

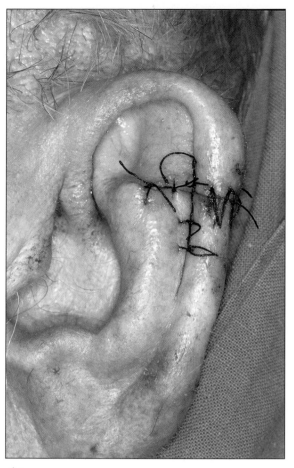

(a)   (b)

Figure 8.9
Wedge excision. This shows wedge excision of a tumour on the helical rim with modification to allow the springy cartilage to close satisfactorily (a). The result after suturing is shown in (b).

Wedge excision of lip, lid and ear

On the margins of the eyelid, lip and ear tumours can be removed by excising a full-thickness wedge or segment-shaped piece containing the tumour and a margin of uninvolved skin. The different tissues contained in the remaining edges are then sutured together to reconstruct the tissue margin. The inherent tissue elasticity of the eyelid and lip enables considerable defects to be repaired in this way without distorting the free margin. On the lip defects smaller than a third of the lip length can be closed directly with a wedge excision, if necessary using a W-plasty correction on the lower lip to avoid excessive distortion. On the eyelid defects of up to 50% can be closed with a direct closure provided the correct design is used. Occasionally a relaxing incision at the corner of the eye is required to increase mobility. Wedge excisions on the ear reduce the ear size and buckling of the ear may occur unless the design is modified to avoid this (Figure 8.9). Ears of different sizes are rarely noticed and for most patients this is not a cosmetic problem. The essential function of the external ear as a support for glasses is not jeopardized by such a procedure.

Wound healing

Open-wound healing

If the wound edges cannot easily be brought together another approach to consider is secondary-intention healing. The wound heals by granulation, contraction and epithelialization – the time taken depending on factors such as the wound site, size and the age of the patient. It is not an all-or-nothing approach and it may be better to close a wound as much as possible without undue tension (leaving the rest to heal by secondary intention) rather than to risk wound-edge necrosis by pulling it too tight. Most wounds allowed to heal by this method do well over time. The contractile forces will inevitably pull on free edges such as the lower eyelid or lip making these areas less suitable for open-wound healing. The cosmetic result of wounds healed by secondary intention varies according to anatomic site (Figure 8.10). Healed wounds are often imperceptible in NEET areas (concave surfaces of the nose, eye, ear and temple). In NOCH areas (convex surfaces of the nose, oral lips, cheeks and chin, and helix of the ear) superficial wounds heal with an acceptable appearance, but deep wounds heal with

depressed or hypertrophic scars acceptable only to some patients. Wounds healed in FAIR areas (forehead, anthelix, eyelids, and remainder of the nose, lips and cheeks) result in flat hypopigmented scars acceptable to many patients. A clinical example of an acceptable result is shown in Figure 8.11. The advantages of secondary-intention healing are that

- it is simple,
- it avoids the need for reconstruction,
- it has a low complication rate,
- recurrences are not buried under flaps or grafts,
- it usually has good cosmetic results.

The disadvantages are that:

- wounds take longer to heal
- there is an increased incidence of hypertrophic scarring,
- it may cause retraction at free edges, for example, lips and eyelids.

Wound care for open-wound healing

Haemostasis must be good. Guiding sutures may be used to form an axis for the wound perpendicular to a free edge such as the lip. It should be cleaned daily with sterile water or a topical antiseptic and then packed with paraffin gauze or filled with an alginate such as Sorbsan. It can then be covered with absorbent gauze. Pressure dressings are invaluable and can lead to better healing with a low complication rate.

Micrographic surgery (Mohs' technique)

Introduction

In the 1940s Fred Mohs, a general surgeon, first described his method of completely excis-

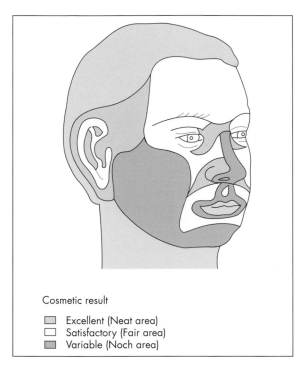

Cosmetic result

▢ Excellent (Neat area)
▢ Satisfactory (Fair area)
▨ Variable (Noch area)

Figure 8.10
The cosmetic results of secondary intention wound healing in different parts of the face.

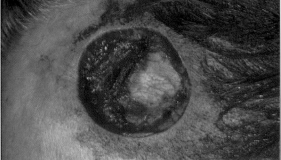

(a)

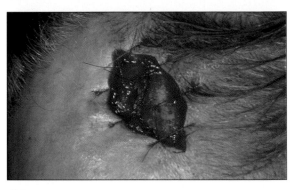

(b)

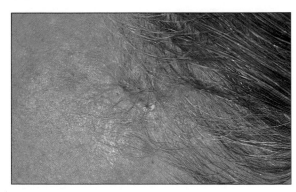

(c)

Figure 8.11
Open wound healing. A wound on the temple (a) is partially closed (b) and left to heal by secondary intention. The result after 4 months showing good preservation of anatomy and acceptable skin texture is shown in (c).

ing recurrent, incompletely excised, poorly defined, histologically aggressive, large or critically sited BCCs. This technique is a common sense way of ensuring complete removal of a tumour that spreads by direct extension. Mohs made the pivotal observation that, in order to be sure that all the tumour was excised, the entire excision margin, and not just selected vertical sections, needed to be examined. He did this by taking horizontal rather than vertical sections so that the complete excision margin was examined. In order to get pieces small enough to be processed and examined the excised skin had to be cut into pieces and thus a map was required so that the original position of each piece could be identified later on the patient's wound.

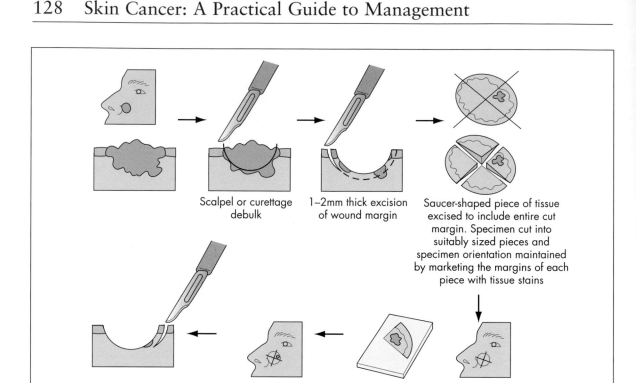

Figure 8.12

Management of difficult skin tumours using micrographic surgery (Mohs' surgery). The clinically evident tumour is first removed by excision or curettage (the debulking stage). A slice of skin 1–2 mm thick is then excised around the edge and deep margin of the wound. This piece of skin has to be cut up into smaller pieces to be histologically processed. Each piece is treated separately and sectioned horizontally so that the entire excision margin is examined. The wound and specimen have to be carefully marked so that the site of each piece can be identified. If tumour is present in one or some of the specimens further excisions are performed until there is no visible tumour at the excision margins. The wound then has to be closed as necessary. (Reproduced with permission from Lawrence C (1996) *An Introduction to Dermatological Surgery* (Blackwell Science: Oxford).)

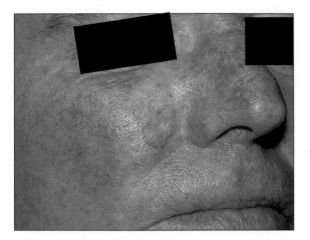

(a)

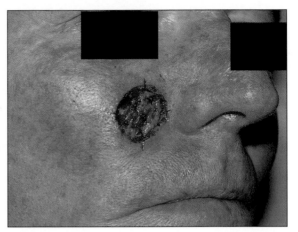

(b)

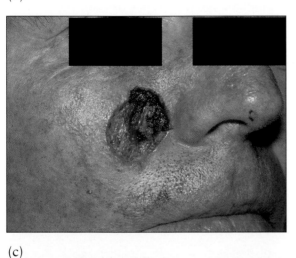

(c)

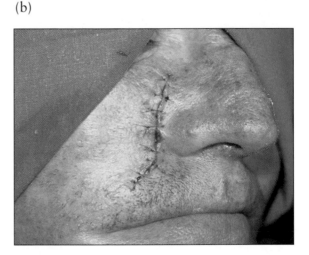

(d)

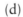

(e)

Figure 8.13
Recurrent BCC. This ill-defined basal cell
carcinoma (a) was excised using Mohs'
horizontal type sections for histological
control. After the first excision (b) there was
still tumour present at the top right excision
margin and this area was therefore re-excised
(c). When it was confirmed that the tumour
had been completely removed the resulting
defect was closed using a cheek advancement
flap (d). By placing the closure line in the
cosmetic boundary between the nose and the
cheek it was less noticeable when seen at
6 months (e).

Table 8.2
Patient information sheet after suture surgery

Your wound has been sutured and it may be tender in 1–2 hours' time when the effect of the local anaesthetic wears off. Leave the dressing in place for at least 24 hours or longer if advised to do so. Rest the area. Avoid strenuous exertion for 48 hours. If the wound bleeds press firmly and directly over it for at least 20 minutes. If bleeding continues seek further medical advice.

Keep the area dry for at least 48 hours. Thereafter you should wash, clean, dry and redress the wound. If the wound is painful take paracetamol rather than aspirin since this may encourage bleeding. If you already take aspirin regularly tell your doctor who will advise whether you need to stop it.

Smoking delays healing. Try to avoid smoking until your stitches are removed.

The pain will start to subside after 2–3 days. If the wound becomes increasingly painful after 3 or 4 days contact the doctor earlier as this may indicate infection.

Your stitches will be removed 4–12 days after surgery, depending on the site and nature of the operation. Ensure that you are going to be available for stitch removal before agreeing to surgery.

Avoid strenuous exertion or activity until your stitches are removed and for some time after suture removal.

Once healed the scar may be red and slightly raised, after several months it will settle to a more flesh-coloured, flat scar.

Technique

Any visible tumour is first removed or debulked by excision or curettage (Figure 8.12). This material is examined histologically but it is not used to determine the adequacy of the excision. The remaining entire wound surface is then excised as a saucer-shaped piece of skin approximately 2 mm thick. This is cut into smaller pieces to facilitate histological processing. The points where it has been divided are marked on the wound and a map is drawn so that the original position of each piece can be identified on the wound. The pieces of skin are then histo-logically examined using horizontal sections so that the entire excision margin is inspected. If residual tumour is identified in a section that portion of the wound is re-excised. The process is repeated until no further tumour is seen. The excised pieces of skin can be prepared for histological examination using in-situ fixation, or in-vitro formalin or fresh frozen tissue fixation. It was the development of the fresh frozen tissue technique in the 1970s that resulted in the widespread adoption of the Mohs' technique because this meant that all the excision stages and the closure could be completed in one day (Figure 8.13).

Wound closure after Mohs' surgery

Once the tumour has been excised the wound closure is managed by either direct closure, flap repair, grafting or secondary-intention healing. When Mohs first described his technique he used in situ tissue fixation using an irritant chemical preparation applied onto the wound. After tumour excision the presence of this material on the skin made closure difficult and he therefore allowed the majority of his earlier wounds to heal by second intention. Whilst second intention healing gives amazingly good results at many sites[5] there are limitations to its use. In the minds of many surgeons not fully familiar with the Mohs' technique the method is incorrectly believed to be synonymous with second-intention healing. In current practice the majority of wounds resulting from micrographic surgery are closed immediately and the various methods used to do this have been discussed.

Postoperative information for patients

Many patients will never have had skin surgery before and will not know what to expect after surgery and prior to suture removal. An information leaflet is helpful and should contain the type of information outlined in Table 8.2.

References

1. Skouge JW (1991) *Skin Grafting*, Practical Manuals in Dermatologic Surgery (Churchill Livingstone: New York).
2. Rohrer TE, Dzubow LM (1995) Conchal bowl skin grafting in nasal tip reconstruction: clinical and histological evaluation, *J Am Acad Dermatol* 33:476–81.
3. Hambley RM, Carruthers JA (1994) Microlipoinjection for the elevation of depressed full thickness grafts on the nose, *J Dermatol Surg Oncol* 20:205–8.
4. Summers BK, Siegle RJ (1993) Facial cutaneous reconstructive surgery. Facial flaps, *J Am Acad Dermatol* 29:917–41.
5. Lawrence CM, Dahl MGC, Comaish JS (1986) Excision of skin malignancies without wound closure, *Br J Dermatol* 115:563–71.

Bibliography

Salasche SJ, Grabski WJ (1990) *Flaps for the Central Face* (Churchill Livingstone: New York).

Salasche SJ, Grabski WJ (1991) Complications of flaps, *J Dermatol Surg Oncol* 17:132–40.

Tebbetts JB (1982) Auricular reconstruction; selected single stage techniques, *J Dermatol Surg Oncol* 8:557–66.

9 Treatment 3 – adjuvant treatment for advanced disease

Basal cell carcinoma

Cure rates for basal cell carcinoma (BCC) decline with each successive attempted therapy and certain features may help to predict which tumours will recur. In 1973 Jackson and Adams defined such characteristics: size of more than 3 cm, local invasion of vital structures, recurrence despite four previous treatments and metastatic spread.[1] Advanced tumours are more common in the elderly and aggressive treatment may not be suitable. However sometimes the situation evolves very slowly and no one on the medical team defines the point at which the BCC is deemed to be advanced. There is some merit in using the American Joint Committee on Cancer (AJCC) TNM (T = tumour, N = lymph node, M = distant metastases) staging system for carcinoma of the skin to define the stage and allow comparison of tumours for inclusion in clinical trials (see Table 9.1).

Dangerously advanced BCC are not common and there is little good comparative evidence to recommend any particular regimen. Using a combination of surgery and radiotherapy 5-year cure rates for T2, T3, and T4 tumours were 93%, 83% and 54% respectively. Most authorities now tend to use combination therapy for T4 tumours. It was once thought that involvement of bone or cartilage precluded the use of radiotherapy but that is no longer the case because tumour

Table 9.1
AJCC TNM staging system.

Primary tumour

T1	2 cm or less greatest dimension
T2	2–5 cm greatest dimension
T3	> 5 cm greatest dimension
T4	Invading deeply, for example, cartilage, muscle, bone

BCC staging

Stage	Tumour	Nodes	Metastasis
I	T1	no	no
II	T2	no	no
	T3	no	no
III	T4	no	no
	T any	yes	no
IV	T any	yes	yes

control is paramount. Fractionated treatments over 6–8 weeks delivering around 6500 cGy is recommended.

Metastatic disease

There are so few cases that no proper trials can be done. If disease has only spread to the local nodes then surgery is indicated, either removing the clinically involved nodes or a block dissection. Most experts have also recommended adjunctive radiotherapy. If the disease has spread to distant sites then surgery may be less feasible but where possible the same principles should apply. However chemotherapy might also be indicated and in this context the agent which has received the most attention is cisplatin being used in monthly cycles.

Squamous cell carcinoma

The staging system for squamous cell carcinoma (SCC) is the same as for BCC in the previous section. Primary tumours which are T2, T3 or T4 can be difficult to cure and careful pre-operative assessment is needed. Clinical examination of draining lymph glands and imaging of the tumour and glands are helpful. Magnetic resonance imaging is the best investigation for determining the extent of soft tissue involvement and the presence of perineural invasion. CT, however, is better for detecting bone and lymph gland involvement. The management of high-risk SCC was discussed in Chapter 4. Postoperative radiation therapy is sometimes used and there is some evidence that local recurrence rates can be reduced.

Managing the neck

Advanced SCC rarely spreads via the blood but readily travels through lymph vessels. The head and neck are common sites for SCC and management of advanced disease in these sites poses several problems. There are complex chains of glands draining the head and neck and some cross channels between them. The problem of how to manage the clinically and/or radiologically disease-free neck is challenging. It has been postulated that if the chance of occult metastasis is 20% or more then treatment is indicated. Radiation therapy and neck dissection give comparable results.[2]

The supraomohyoid method is not too aggressive and if these nodes are clear it is most unlikely that the other chains are involved. If intra-operative frozen sections reveal tumour it is possible to progress to the modified radical neck dissection. If later reports show tumour in more than one node then adjuvant radiotherapy may be used.

Management strategies for the clinically involved neck glands derive from the experience of maxillo-facial surgeons working with tumours of the oropharynx. Where multiple glands or extracapsular spread is found neck dissection with adjuvant radiotherapy is generally recommended.

Chemotherapy

Several agents have been tried for patients with advanced SCC. Cisplatin, doxorubicin, 5-fluorouracil and bleomycin individually or in combination have been beneficial giving complete remission for up to 3 years. Usually chemotherapy is given before or after the definitive treatment of surgery or radiotherapy. The numbers involved in these studies are not large enough to produce a strong evidence base but there seems to be enough benefit to warrant further efforts in this direction to control advanced SCC of the skin.

Biological response modifiers

Small studies involving retinoids and interferon-alpha have given benefit to patients with relatively minor side-effects. High doses of either drug are more toxic and the role of these therapies is still being assessed.

Malignant melanoma

Interferon alpha

Interferon alpha 2a and 2b have been used to treat melanoma for over 15 years, both as adjuvant treatment in apparently disease-free patients, and in patients with metastatic disease. In the latter setting it appears to have little value, but interest has increased in its use as adjuvant treatment following surgery for primary or loco-regional disease. There are 10 published studies describing its use, and of these three appear to show benefit. The first is ECOG 1684. This trial randomized 287 patients, mainly those with treated lymph node recurrence, to receive either high-dose interferon alpha 2b for 1 year, or observation. After 6.9 years of follow-up there appeared to be a small difference in outcome in favour of the interferon-treated group. Of patients treated with interferon, 81 out of 142 had died compared with 90 out of 137 patients in the observation group. Although the trial was well designed and executed, toxicity from this regime was serious; 67% had grade 3 or more toxicity and 50% of the patients required dose reductions or delays during treatment. The therapeutic benefit appeared so small that many remained sceptical, although the drug was licensed for use in melanoma both in the USA in 1996 and then in the UK in 1997. However, a study designed to further compare this treatment with low-dose interferon and with observation (ECOG 1690) has not confirmed the original findings, with no survival benefit from high-dose interferon.

High- or intermediate-dose interferon alpha 2b is still the subject of two trials despite the unpromising data discussed above. EORTC 18952 investigated intermediate doses on the basis that this was what patients could actually tolerate in the two ECOG studies. Recruitment finished in 2000, and preliminary results should be available in 2002. EORTC 18991 is another very large randomized control trial comparing a modified form of interferon alpha 2b. By attaching it to polyethylene glycol, pegylated or PEG-Intron has the advantage of reduced frequency of injections – once weekly – and less toxicity. The trial opens in 2000, and should complete accrual over 24 months.

Preliminary data from two studies of low-dose interferon alpha 2a appear to show small increases in disease-free survival but this may not translate into increased overall survival. Further data from these trials are awaited, together with the findings of the UKCCCR-sponsored trial of low-dose interferon (AIM High), which compares 3 MU of interferon alpha 2a with observation in patients with primary melanoma 4 mm or more, or loco-regional metastasis. Preliminary data from this trial should be available by 2002. Interferon, even in low dosage, is a toxic drug. Flu-like symptoms are common, and the associated malaise, tiredness and depression can seriously reduce quality of life. Myelosuppression and abnormal liver function tests are also fairly common but these effects are usually mild and recovery is quick on drug withdrawal. In high-doses, toxicity can be life threatening. Interferon is awkward to use, since it needs to be given by injection three times weekly. Despite the inadequacy of the evidence for benefit, interferon alpha 2a was licensed in the UK in 1999 for use in melanoma. However, the uncertainty about its value and its toxicity mean that it is still an experimental drug in this context.

Vaccines

Interest in melanoma vaccines has increased recently. There is evidence for efficacy in metastatic disease and preliminary evidence for adjuvant vaccine treatment. However, melanoma immunotherapy is in its infancy and there are many vaccines targeting a variety of epitopes by different means so that it is difficult to establish which approaches hold promise. The use of peptide-pulsed dendritic cells to present antigens to T cells is particularly interesting but it is likely that, as with interferon, large trials will be needed to discover whether such treatments work. The EORTC will launch their trial of adjuvant GM2 vaccine in melanoma in mid 2000, and this will recruit 1200 patients with primary melanoma of 1.5 mm or more over an estimated 3 years. Consequently, as with interferon these are still investigative treatments. Patients who wish to consider adjuvant drug treatment should be referred to a centre which participates in melanoma clinical trials.

Radiotherapy

Adjuvant radiotherapy has a well-defined place in melanoma. The best evidence is from head and neck melanoma, where radiotherapy following neck dissection for lymph node metastasis significantly reduces the risk of further recurrence in the neck. The evidence for its use elsewhere is less clear, but a good case could be made for treating extensive recurrence in other nodal basins following block dissection. For instance, very large (5 cm or more) lymph nodes and/or large numbers of nodes (five or more) with extra capsular spread in an axilla could represent a significant risk for subsequent relapse and local morbidity, for example, with brachial plexus involvement. Adjuvant radiotherapy may well reduce that risk, although it clearly does have morbidity of its own and in particular can make lymphoedema worse. One of the most difficult problems in melanoma

is the patient with progressive loco-regional disease but no distant metastases. It is always worth bearing in mind the potential benefit of aggressive local treatment.

Isolated limb perfusion

Adjuvant treatment with regional chemotherapy for primary limb melanoma has been shown to be ineffective. However, loco-regional recurrence in a limb may take several forms. The first, and most common, is simply a hard 1–2 cm subcutaneous lump. Provided these can be excised completely, they should present no further problem. Dermal papules and nodules 1 mm and upwards are often multiple, superficial, and can be treated with electrosurgery or carbon dioxide laser destruction. However this condition is usually progressive and treatment may need to be repeated every 2–3 months. Eventually it may begin to involve deeper structures in and below muscle fascia. There will be pain and induration and if it extends into the vasculature or bone the limb is under threat. Isolated limb perfusion is a means of delivering high-dose local chemotherapy to the limb but it is an invasive technique. It requires isolation of the circulation of the limb with cannulation of the vessels in the groin or axilla followed by perfusion with Melphalan or tumour necrosis factor through the oxygenated hyperthermic limb for up to 1 h. Tumours begin to shrink over 2–3 weeks, but responses may not be complete for several months. About 40% of patients have a complete response, another 40% partial regression but 20% do not respond. Risks include postoperative compartment syndrome, arterial thrombosis and limb loss. Isolated limb infusion is a recent development and appears similar in efficacy, but is safer and cheaper.

Alternative (complementary) therapy (immune system, diets, positive thinking)

There is little published work on the role of alternative medicine in the management of nonmelanoma skin cancer. Perhaps because melanoma is a life-threatening disease patients are motivated to become involved in their treatment and more has been written on the subject. A Gerson's or lactovegetarian diet with low sodium, fat and protein but high potassium, fluid and nutrients was used in patients with advanced melanoma. Almost twice as many of the 153 patients who used this diet survived to 5 years compared to the results from other melanoma studies.[3] It is of course impossible to judge the true value of such treatments in terms of survival without properly conducted and controlled comparisons. However, this study suggests that such an investigation is merited. Patients faced with the knowledge that they have advanced melanoma may feel helpless. Such patients recognize that nonconventional therapies are supplementary to standard medical treatment but may draw strength from them because they provide a way of avoiding passivity and coping with feelings of hopelessness.[4]

References

1. Jackson R, Adams RH (1973) Horrifying basal cell carcinoma; a study of 33 cases and a comparison with 435 nonhorror cases and a report on 4 metastatic cases, *J Surg Oncol* 5:431–63.
2. Weiss MH, Harrison LB, Isaacs RS (1994) Use of decision analysis in planning a management strategy in the N0 neck, *Arch Otolaryngol Head Neck Surg* 120:699–702.
3. Hildenbrand GL, Hildenbrand LC, Bradford K et al (1995) 5 Year survival rates of melanoma patients treated by diet therapy after the manner of Gerson: a retrospective review, *Altern Ther Health Med* 1:29–37.
4. Sollner W, Zing-Schir M, Rumpold G et al (1997) Attitude toward alternative therapy, compliance with standard treatment and the need for emotional support in patients with melanoma, *Arch Dermatol* 133:316–21.

10 Prevention and education

Introduction

The role of a public health service is to promote healthy living in order to limit the development of disease within the population as a whole. To do this requires involvement not only of the health services but also of government agencies at both a national and local level. Historically infectious diseases were the major causes of disease and death and early public health measures were aimed at their control. Although the fight against infectious disease is by no means won, their impact on health in the developed world has been dramatically reduced. Conditions such as cardiovascular disease and cancer have replaced the infectious diseases as the major causes of ill health and death.

Skin cancer is the most common form of cancer found worldwide in light-skinned people. The incidence of skin cancer is increasing at an alarming rate. It has been estimated that the incidence of nonmelanoma skin cancer is increasing at 5% per annum in the UK. The recent dramatic increase in the incidence of melanoma appears to be slowing but it causes the majority of the deaths due to skin cancer. Although the mortality associated with skin cancer, including melanoma, is lower than that for many other cancers, melanoma accounts for more years of life lost per case than any other cancer, including cancer of the breast and lung. In addition skin cancer causes a significant degree of morbidity and places a large burden on healthcare providers. This makes the reduction in the incidence of skin cancer a major goal for public health prevention programmes.

To prevent the development of skin cancer is a more complicated task than the control of infectious diseases. This is due to the long latent period between exposure and development of the cancer. In addition this is complicated by the fact that the true role of the various putative aetiological agents has not been fully elucidated, especially for melanoma. It is not simply a matter of introducing a variety of environmental or social initiatives to reduce exposure of the population to the causative factor.

To prevent skin cancer may need a change in behaviour and lifestyle at a time in people's lives when the risk seems remote. To change behaviour requires education to improve understanding and knowledge of the disease. Health education alone is not always sufficient to achieve this goal. Health promotion is a complex process that involves empowerment of the whole population in improving its health through education, the provision of preventative services and improving the environment. It requires political advocacy as well as the energy and determination of the health services.

The earliest efforts at prevention of skin cancer were set up in Australia by clinicians concerned with their experience of an increasing incidence of melanoma. These early campaigns, started in the mid 1960s, were health education initiatives.

By the early 1970s the concept of the New Public Health was developed in Canada. This incorporated health promotion as a vital component of any initiative aimed at improving public health. Health promotion involves the healthcare providers, experts in education, social services and environmental planners. The 'First International Conference on Health Promotion' was held in Ottawa in 1986 and agreed a charter outlining the key components of health promotion campaigns. These principles have been adopted by many countries around the world. The World Health Organization outlined the concept of 'Health for All by the year 2000' at the International Conference on Primary Health Care at Alma-Ata in 1978.[1] This suggested that health policy makers in each country should set health targets by which their efforts could be monitored. Many countries have set such targets, and utilizing the principles of health promotion, are attempting to improve the quality of health of their populations. In the UK in 1992 the then Conservative government passed the white paper 'The Health of the Nation'.[2] This white paper set out the target for skin cancer 'to halt the year-on-year increase in the incidence of skin cancers by 2005'. The new Labour government has maintained this commitment in its 1999 white paper 'Saving Lives: Our Healthier Nation'.[3]

- primary prevention – to prevent a disease process starting,
- secondary prevention – to detect disease at an early, curable stage and institute effective treatment,
- tertiary prevention – for 'damage limitation' in people with established disease.

Skin cancer is the result of the complex interaction between the host with a predetermined susceptibility, his or her behaviour and environmental factors. In health the balance of these forces favours the host. If this balance is altered either by changes in host susceptibility, their behaviour or changes in the environment, skin cancer will result. Prevention of these cancers requires effective intervention in the dynamic relationship of the above factors to restore the healthy balance.

The increase in skin cancer during the latter half of the twentieth century suggests a major role for an environmental factor in the pathogenesis of the disease. It is not essential that the precise cause of a disease is known for preventive action to be successful. Exposure to ultraviolet radiation in sunlight has been identified as the most likely, but by no means certain culprit. As the understanding of the pathogenesis of skin cancer has increased it has become apparent that the different forms have different relationships to sun exposure. This has led to mixed messages being delivered on sun avoidance and this lack of clarity has caused confusion within the public at large. Therefore to enable effective prevention campaigns to be developed, it is imperative that the pathogenesis of each of the major types of skin cancer is elucidated.

Principles of prevention

Preventive action has been classified into the following strategies:

Changing behaviour

Most public health measures for prevention of skin cancer are aimed at altering the behaviour of individuals. Primary prevention is attempted by promoting sun protection and sun avoidance with various public education campaigns. Secondary prevention is achieved by increasing public awareness in reporting suspicious lesions early, while still at a curable stage.

Sun avoidance

The message that skin cancer is caused by overexposure to solar ultraviolet radiation appears simple and should cause individuals to limit their sun exposure so reducing the incidence of skin cancer. Unfortunately, for a variety of reasons this view is too simplistic. The relationship between skin cancer and sun exposure is complex. Of the three main types of skin cancer it is only squamous cell carcinoma (SCC) that appears to be directly related to the total cumulative sun exposure in an individual's lifetime.[4] Sun avoidance at any stage in life will therefore delay the development of SCC. Reduction of the total ultraviolet exposure by 50% would theoretically double the age at which SCC develop and for most individuals this would make the disease irrelevant as they would be well past their 100th birthday!

In contrast, melanoma[5] and possibly also basal cell carcinoma (BCC),[6] appear to be related to intermittent high-intensity exposure to sunlight, especially if received in the first 10 years of life. The need to protect young children and limit subsequent episodes of sunburn is thus far more important than the complete avoidance of sun exposure for melanoma prevention. This has led to the confusing concept of a 'safe tan' which may offer protection to the subsequent development of melanoma. Evidence to support this concept is not conclusive although it may help

explain the fact that people who work outside are at lower risk of melanoma than people who only have recreational exposure to the sun. It is also recognized that the ability to develop a suntan easily is a phenotypic marker of a reduced susceptibility to develop melanoma as opposed to being protective in its own right.

To effectively convey the message that sun exposure is harmful you first have to understand why people seek the sun and have the perception of a suntan being a desirable characteristic. This phenomenon is relatively recent and dates from the early part of the twentieth century. The advent of the industrial revolution caused the working classes to spend most of their working lives in the sunless environment of the factory, mill or coal mine. The financial ability to travel and the use of heliotherapy for the treatment of tuberculosis caused the sun tan to become a marker of wealth and health. More recently the recognition of seasonal affective disorder being related to ambient levels of sunlight may also have added happiness to this equation. The effects of the cinema and the fashion industry together with the advent of the consumer-led society has greatly enhanced this positive image of the suntan. In the short space of 50–60 years we have witnessed a complete reversal in behaviour. People once actively avoided the sun, by wearing protective clothing and resting during the hottest and brightest part of the day. Now it seems many people take every possible opportunity to chase, and then expose themselves to, the sun. This means that not only do people get positive reinforcement from being in the sun but there are also huge commercial pressures to maintain this situation. The fight to reverse this trend has not been helped by the variety of and occasionally contradictory messages that have been delivered by health professionals themselves.

For health promotion initiatives to change behaviour they need to tackle the need to reduce sun exposure at both the individual level as well as in society as a whole. At the individual level health promotion campaigns can attempt to increase awareness of the dangers of sun exposure. When concerned specifically with melanoma prevention it is imperative that this message is delivered to parents of young children and also the children themselves. There is evidence to suggest that the most effective time to deliver this message to children is between the ages of eight and ten. The children need to be old enough to appreciate the nature of the message but young enough that they have not already developed detrimental behavioural patterns. To try and achieve this a variety of education packages have been used to raise knowledge and ultimately to influence behaviour in school children. It appears that course work spread over weeks involving lectures, videos and interactive and project work are more effective than isolated lectures. This is obviously resource intensive but as it involves doing work at home it has the added advantage of being an effective method for delivering the message to the parents as well.[7]

In conjunction with these programmes to raise knowledge within the school environment it is also necessary to reinforce the message to the wider population via media campaigns. Unfortunately, when dealing with older individuals they often have established patterns of behaviour which have to be altered. Individuals will have a psychological conflict in deciding between their desire for a suntan and the message that this will cause them harm. In this situation people will often deny the risk, or perceive the risk as being so small that the development of a tan outweighs it. Other people while admitting that there is a risk from sun exposure find that the use of sun protection is either too cumbersome or is cosmetically unacceptable. In this situation promoting a sun avoidance message in an alternative way may be more effective whilst playing on other fears may be justified. It is true to say that people who have a high regard for their physical appearance are more likely to desire a suntan. For these individuals stressing the photoageing properties of the UVA rays in sunshine (and from tanning lamps), that 'this year's sun tan is next year's wrinkle', may cause more concern than the long-term cancer risk. Another way to increase the perception of risk from the sun is to utilize people's fear of passivity. If it is purely a personal decision on whether to take a risk or not, individuals can easily minimize or deny this risk. If however you 'impose' an additional risk on them this can assume sinister proportions. This has been seen with the fear of passive smoking which has led to banning of smoking in many public institutions and transport services. In the fight against sun exposure, the reduction in the ozone layer and the subsequent increase in levels of ultraviolet radiation reaching the earth's surface can be used as an additional spur for people to change established behaviour.

It does appear that these campaigns have increased the knowledge of skin cancer and the risks of sun exposure within the general public. Unfortunately it has been more difficult to demonstrate a marked change in behaviour. Interestingly, there has been a slow change in the attitude of the media, advertising and the fashion industry to the tan. The cosmetic industry has seen this as a commercial opportunity and are now promoting sun protection and anti-ageing products together. At the time of writing this has even entered the realm of popular culture. This slow drift away from the positive perception of the tan may ultimately have a greater effect on behaviour.

Sunscreens

Health promotion campaigns often concentrate on promoting sun protection, that is, the use of sunscreens, hats and sunglasses as in the 'slip! slop! slap!' campaign in Australia or sun avoidance as in the UK 'shift to the shade' campaign. Unfortunately certain aspects of these campaigns have caused controversy so diluting the message; this has particularly been seen with the use of sunscreens.

Sunscreens were initially designed as tanning aids; by blocking the burning UVB rays they enabled people to stay in the sun for longer and thus achieve a tan more quickly without the pain of sunburn. As such they were sold as cosmetics with marketing to match. As both the ageing effects of UVA radiation and the cancer risk of sun exposure became more apparent, so sunscreens have changed. It is important to understand how sunscreens work to enable sensible advice to be given on their use. Sunscreens are composed of either colourless organic compounds which absorb ultraviolet radiation and so render it ineffective, or inorganic compounds which reflect or scatter the ultraviolet radiation. The majority of older sunscreens were effective at absorbing UVB radiation but they required the incorporation of reflecting compounds to block UVA radiation which rendered them cosmetically unacceptable. Recently new UVA-absorbing compounds have been developed and incorporated into sunblocks so that broad-spectrum screens are now available to protect against both UVA and UVB radiation.

The sun protection factor (SPF) of a sunscreen relates to the ability of the agent to lengthen the time to induce erythema or sunburn. Thus the use of a sunscreen with an SPF of 2 means that an individual will take twice as long to become sunburnt. The wavelength dependence for solar erythema is within the UVB spectrum, therefore the SPF rating of a sunscreen only relates to its ability to block UVB radiation and not to its UVA-blocking characteristics. More recently a variety of methods have been developed to grade the degree of UVA protection. This is indicated by a star system in the UK. For a sunscreen to perform to its marketed standard it needs to be applied evenly to all sun-exposed areas. On an average adult approximately 50–60 ml of product is required. If used properly it means there are only three full applications per standard bottle. In reality if people do use a sunscreen they apply it much more sparingly than this, which dramatically reduces the effectiveness of the protection.

Although sunscreens can protect against the acute effects of sun exposure, controversy still exists over whether they can prevent skin cancer. There is evidence to show that sunscreens can prospectively prevent dysplastic changes such as the development of actinic keratoses.[8] Animal models have shown that they can protect against the development of certain skin cancers but notably not melanoma or BCC. Indeed more worryingly there is some evidence to show that the use of sunscreens actually increases the risk of development of melanoma.[9] It is vitally important that this observation is clarified. Certainly recall bias may account for some of this discrepancy. More importantly however, there is evidence that the use of sunscreens may paradoxically increase exposure to the more dangerous part of the ultraviolet spectrum for the development of melanoma. The role of UVA radiation in the production of melanoma is gaining interest. To date the evidence supporting this is derived indirectly. If UVA exposure is important, the way people use their sunblocks will have to change. People still tend to use sunblocks to lengthen their stay in the sun without getting a sunburn. Thus they actually are exposed to more of the dangerous UVA radiation. Until more is known about the action spectrum for the production of all types of skin cancer, sunscreens cannot be promoted as protective against skin cancer when used alone. It is more prudent to promote the use of sunscreens as one part of a sensible approach to sun protection together with suitable clothing and sensible behaviour. They certainly should not be used to increase the length of time spent in the sun, and if used need to be applied consistently and effectively. Broad-spectrum blocks are preferable to those that primarily protect against UVB radiation.

The use of clothing provides a simple but very effective method for reducing sun exposure. In general clothing which is thicker and has a tighter weave is better at blocking ultraviolet radiation.[10] The amount of ultraviolet radiation that can penetrate a particular article of clothing depends not only on the material and weave but also on whether it is wet or dry. It is now possible to purchase clothing which is designed to be ultraviolet protective when wet. Clothing can now be graded with an ultraviolet protection factor (UPF), this is analogous to an SPF marking. A T-shirt with a UPF of 10 would afford the same level of protection as a sunblock with an SPF of 10; in practice however the T-shirt is more effective as it performs as the stated UPF to all areas that it covers.

Hats are another useful accessory that provide shade to the face. They can dramatically reduce direct ultraviolet radiation from the sun although they work less well for reflected rays from water surfaces.

Sunbeds

The continuing perception that a tan is synonymous with good health accounts for the continuing popularity of tanning devices. These devices can be found in solariums on any high street and are increasingly being found in leisure complexes and health clubs. Smaller portable devices can also be found within the home. The term 'tanorexia' has recently been coined to describe individuals living in temperate climates who appear to be addicted to the use of sunbeds more than once a week, all year round, to achieve a permanent tan. These individuals are receiving 'extra' ultraviolet radiation which is the equivalent of living in the tropics where the incidence of skin cancer is eight-fold that of people living in temperate climates.

The older devices emitted predominantly UVB radiation which, as well as delivering a tan, could also cause extensive and painful burns if used incorrectly. New devices emit predominantly UVA radiation and are being marketed as providing a tan safely. As our knowledge grows about the causes of photoageing and the action spectrum for carcinogenesis widens it is realized that these devices cannot be used without risk. It has now been demonstrated that exposure to 10 sessions per year under a tanning lamp increases the risk of developing all forms of skin cancer. This has prompted calls for legislation to regulate the use of these lamps and for local authorities to remove these devices from their leisure facilities. Unfortunately their use is so widespread that this may force people to seek facilities in establishments where it would not be possible to monitor the safety of equipment. Equipment in commercially run tanning parlours has been shown to vary widely with regard to the amount of energy produced and also the spectrum of the emission, with significant amounts of the more dangerous UVB being emitted from many lamps.[11]

In 1991 the International Radiation Protection Organization (IRPO) and the International Non-Ionizing Radiation Committee (INIRC) issued guidelines on the use of tanning devices. They stated that their use for cosmetic purposes could not be generally recommended. They also issued specific recommendations against their use by people with skin types I and II, people with a large number of moles and people with evidence of chronic sun damage or who have had either premalignant or malignant skin lesions. They also specifically warned against their use by children. The British Photobiology Group's recommendations broadly follows these guidelines. However if people are determined to use a tanning device they recommend that use should be limited to two courses per year and that each course should consist of no more than 10 sessions.

Legislative changes

The majority of health promotion campaigns aim to change behaviour at an individual level. Unfortunately although public knowledge has undoubtedly been increased about the dangers of sun exposure and the risks of skin cancer, this does not always translate into a change in behaviour. On occasions sacrificing free will by introducing legislative changes can have more of an effect on preventing unhealthy habits. The fight against skin cancer could be helped by the introduction of measures to limit sun exposure both in schools and at work. Success with this approach can be seen in the Australian policy of 'no hat – no play' rules at schools. Similar measures could be demanded of people who work outside. In the workplace, occupational exposure to ultraviolet radiation should be limited. Artificial light sources are used in a variety of ways in the work setting, from welding lamps to high-intensity lamps used in crack detection and insecticidal ultra-

violet sources used in the food industry. Health and safety at work legislation demands that employees are protected from overexposure to any ultraviolet radiation from these sources.

Local health authorities could remove sunbeds from their sports and leisure facilities and also could be made to provide covered play areas for children. Measures such as these may seem far fetched particularly in countries with relatively low levels of natural sunshine, such as the UK. However, as well as reinforcing the sun protection message, changes such as these would make it easier for people to adopt a safer lifestyle.

Early detection

Hand in hand with campaigns aimed at changing behaviour to reduce sun exposure and increase the awareness of skin cancer, structures have to be put in place for the early detection and treatment of skin cancers while they are at an easily managed and curable stage. Most efforts at secondary prevention have been aimed exclusively at the early detection of melanoma. This is not only because of its greater metastatic potential but also because the much larger numbers of non-melanoma skin cancers would overwhelm most secondary prevention campaigns.

Screening

Wilson and Junger outlined the requirements for a screening programme to be successful:[12]

- the condition should be an important health problem,
- facilities should be readily available for screening and treatment,

- there should be a recognizable early stage of the disease,
- effective treatment for patients found to have the disease should be available,
- there needs to be an effective screening test or examination,
- the test or examination should be acceptable to the population,
- the pathogenesis and course of the disease should be adequately understood,
- there needs to be an agreed policy on who to treat,
- the economic costs of screening and treatment of people recognized with disease should be balanced when compared to the overall expenditure on health,
- screening should be a continuous process.

In many respects skin cancer, particularly melanoma, fulfils many if not all of these criteria. It is a growing health problem with an increasing mortality which can be recognized by a simple skin examination which is essentially an office-based procedure. Certainly in the case of melanoma, the superficial spreading form goes through a stage where treatment conveys a very good prognosis. Although a skin examination and simple surgical treatments are relatively cheap, the size of the problem and the at-risk population demand a huge investment in time and resources if the whole of the at-risk population were to be periodically screened.

Although institutions such as the American Academy of Dermatology have advocated periodic skin checks on a nationwide basis, to date this has only been on a voluntary basis. Selective screening programmes for melanoma have been carried out in the workplace and also on sunbathers on beaches. Targeting particularly high-risk populations would be a sensible approach if rigorous screening programmes were to be implemented.

Examples of people at particular risk of skin cancer are those with known genetic mutations such as Gorlin's syndrome and xeroderma pigmentosum although these conditions are rare. A larger group of individuals are transplant recipients who are on long-term immunosuppressive therapy and are known to be at a much higher risk of developing skin cancer. To date the response to focused screening has been encouraging. Nevertheless, for the rest of the population at large, screening for melanoma will still be only performed on a voluntary basis for the foreseeable future. In the USA and some European countries this approach has been adopted. In the USA, the American Academy of Dermatology funds melanoma recognition days where free screening for melanoma is offered, but not treatment.

Initiatives like this have proved very popular. Melanomas detected in this fashion tend to be thinner than those from other clinics. This approach is very labour intensive and demands high numbers of dermatologists to staff such screening clinics. A similar approach is neither cost effective nor feasible in countries such as the UK with relatively few dermatologists per capita.

Pigmented lesion clinics

An alternative approach to enable the early recognition of skin cancers, particularly melanoma, is the provision of easy access to a specialist clinic. Here staff and services are fully resourced to detect and subsequently treat early lesions. This approach requires the prior education of other physicians and ultimately the general public in the recognition of the signs of malignancy. Examples of these early diagnosis campaigns have been set up around the world, notably in Queensland,

Australia, Italy and the West of Scotland. From preliminary data collected in these studies it was seen that the predominant reason for delay in treatment of melanoma lay with the patients themselves. Initially professional education campaigns provided primary care physicians with clear instructions and sensitive and specific descriptions of precursor and early thin melanomas. Once this had been achieved the awareness of the population at large was increased with a series of public health education campaigns. These campaigns, delivered via newspaper articles, television and radio broadcasts, aim to increase the awareness of the general public, not only about the dangers of skin cancer but also about the clinical appearance. Television broadcasts have proved to be one of the most effective media for conveying the health education message. This form of approach utilizes pre-existing healthcare systems and referral practices. It can be speeded up by implementing specialized, fast-track clinics but also requires the provision of fast-track surgery. In the UK this has been made possible by the development of pigmented lesion clinics where experienced dermatologists provide a diagnostic service and in close liaison with specialist surgeons access to definitive surgical treatment. This type of clinic requires the co-operation of the local GPs so that it is not abused as a method of obtaining a quick opinion on another less urgent dermatological problem. The introduction of specialist clinics for the early detection of melanoma in Queensland and the West of Scotland resulted in an increase in the proportion of thin, and therefore potentially curable melanomas, particularly in young females. In Italy it appeared to produce a decrease in the expected deaths from melanoma in the male population. The advantages of dedicated pigmented clinics are numerous; not only do

they provide a better pick-up rate than other clinics, they also provide a focus for a multi-disciplinary approach with other clinicians as well as a good educational resource.

Tertiary prevention

Unfortunately metastatic melanoma responds poorly to treatment and so the main thrust of care is towards palliation. For thin melanomas that have been excised the situation is different. A prior history of melanoma is a strong risk factor for the development of further primary tumours, so these patients need to be educated more carefully on the signs and symptoms of early melanoma. Patients with a family history of melanoma and also an atypical mole syndrome phenotype probably warrant long-term follow-up.

The presence of a nonmelanoma skin cancer is also a risk factor for the subsequent development of both melanoma and other nonmelanoma skin cancers. It would not be feasible to follow up all these patients. High-risk patients such as those on long-term immunosuppression or those genetically predisposed to tumours such as patients with Gorlin's syndrome or xeroderma pigmentosum again warrant different follow-up arrangements.

It has been shown that treatment with retinoids can reduce the subsequent development of both premalignant lesions and invasive carcinomas. In this situation the retinoids are temporarily suppressing the expansion of the mutated clone. If treatment is subsequently stopped these clones will start to multiply again and fresh cancers will develop. 5-Fluorouracil is an antimetabolite which may also be used for chemoprevention of nonmelanoma skin cancers. Unlike systemic retinoids, fluorouracil can remove initiated cells and so cause regression of dysplastic clones. The use of retinoids or topical fluorouracil may be considered in these high-risk patients but needs to be weighed against the side-effect profile of these medicines.

Environmental changes

Most efforts at skin cancer prevention have gone towards changing individual behaviour and speeding up the process of diagnosis and treatments. The environment is another area where efforts can be made to reduce the likelihood of cancer development. In 1974 Molina and Rowland predicted that industrially produced halogenated compounds would diffuse into the upper atmosphere and destroy the ozone in the stratosphere.[13] Ten years later it became clear that this prediction was coming true with a so-called ozone hole developing over the Antarctic. Ozone absorbs UVB radiation and concern was expressed that this would ultimately lead to higher levels of ambient ultraviolet radiation reaching the earth's surface, fuelling the increase in incidence of skin cancer.

Despite this it was not until the agreement of the Montreal protocol in 1987 that the developed industrial world agreed to limit the production of these compounds. It took nearly another 10 years before the total production of chlorofluorinated carbons (the major cause of ozone depletion) was finally limited. We can now expect a slow reversal in stratospheric ozone depletion. The ozone story shows that it is possible to override national and commercial interests and to prevent or reverse damage to the global environment. This gives a shred of hope for the future well-being of this planet. The precise role of ultraviolet radiation in the pathogenesis of melanoma is still disputed and a variety of other environmental factors have at various times been implicated as causative agents for melanoma. Water pollution appears to be one factor that deserves more research and if an association is proven, then greater efforts at reducing the levels of these pollutants both at national and international level would be demanded.

At a local level there are changes that can be made to the environment to promote healthier living with respect to sun exposure. Schools and sporting and leisure facilities could be provided with areas of shade. Shade can be constructed either as permanent or semipermanent canopies or awnings, or it can be created naturally by planting broad-leaf trees. It has been estimated that a tree in leaf provides shade equivalent to an SPF of 15. It must be appreciated that shade protects the individual from direct sunshine but not necessarily from reflected light, thus when situated near water surfaces or light flat surfaces such as concrete, additional protection needs to be taken.

Review of prevention campaigns

Health promotion activities are costly in both time and money and it therefore behoves those funding and implementing these services to ensure that they achieve the desired goal of reducing the incidence of, and mortality from, skin cancer. The vast majority of prevention campaigns have been aimed exclusively at melanoma. As has been mentioned, the long latent period between carcinogen exposure and the development of melanoma makes analysis of the success of prevention programmes difficult. There is certainly good evidence that education programmes can improve the knowledge base of the population regarding the dangers of excess sun exposure and skin cancer.[14] Unfortunately it has been harder to demonstrate a sustained change in behaviour. Where changes in behaviour have occurred they are predominantly seen in women and young adults. Following intensive campaigns in Australia there was a three-fold increase in the number of people reporting the use of sunscreen and a similar reduction in the number of reported sunburns. Unfortunately when the actual percentages are taken into account, an increase from 10% to only 28% reporting the use of sunscreen and a reduction from 14% to 5% in reported sunburns, the effects of these campaigns are disappointing. More worryingly these behaviour changes appear to wear off gradually over time.

The effects of the early detection programmes both in Australia and Europe appear to have had a greater impact. Certainly following the introduction of these programmes in Queensland and in the West of Scotland, a reduction in the delay in the presentation of melanomas and the proportion of better prognosis, thin tumours being excised was demonstrated.

These findings are encouraging, however the ultimate success of all prevention campaigns has to be measured in terms of changes in overall mortality from melanoma. Again the data are promising. In the West of Scotland the reduction in delay in presentation of melanoma has also been associated with a fall in mortality from melanoma, especially in women. Across the whole of Europe over the period from 1978 to 1989 there has been an overall increase in survival from melanoma.[15] This is felt to be due to the fact that more thin, good prognosis tumours are now being treated which may reflect earlier reporting of melanoma.

This may not be the only explanation however. Data from Australia have revealed that the age-standardized mortality rates rose steadily in birth cohorts from the mid 1800s until the 1930s. Since then there has been a levelling in mortality rates in subsequent birth cohorts. Thus it could have been predicted that there would be a levelling in overall mortality by the end of the twentieth century irrespective of the introduction of prevention campaigns. The data on European survival rates reveal a marked difference between survival in more developed areas compared with poorer countries in Eastern Europe. The percentage of thicker, poor prognosis tumours is much higher in these countries and can help explain this difference. It has been shown that even after controlling for tumour thickness, socio-economic status is a major factor influencing survival. Thus the general improvement in quality of life through this century and the geographic discrepancies in socio-economic characteristics may also explain certain of these changes in mortality rates and survival that are now being seen. It has been postulated that this is due to the consumption of anti-oxidants and improvements in nutrition which may have a more profound effect on tumour biology.

In the context of skin cancer prevention most of the efforts have been directed at the prevention of melanoma. The increase in nonmelanoma cancers has received little attention to date despite the fact that they place a large burden on health services. Chemoprevention with retinoids has been shown to be effective in certain high-risk groups but the more widespread use of these agents has not been tested.

Agencies co-ordinating protection campaigns in the UK

In the UK, the Secretary of State for Health is responsible to parliament for the promotion and protection of the health of the nation. The Health Education Authority (HEA) is charged with leading and co-ordinating health promotion. The HEA are led by a board made up of leading clinicians, allied healthcare professionals, educationalists and also members of the media. It directly advises the Secretary of State on health promotion matters and helps to formulate health promotion targets. In 1992 the 'Health of the Nation', a strategic policy document, was published. This listed five key areas of health action; one of these areas was cancer and its stated aim for skin cancer was to halt the year-on-year increase in skin cancer by the year 2005.

In addition the HEA has a major role in providing health information to the general public, and also helps other organizations in their efforts to provide health education. In the fight against skin cancer there are many organizations involved at various different levels. The UK Skin Cancer Working Group was established in response to the 'Health of the Nation' document. It acts as a meeting point for agencies concerned with the primary and secondary prevention of skin cancer in the UK. It was set up by the British Association of Dermatologists and has members representing the British Association of Plastic Surgeons, the Imperial Cancer Research Fund, the Cancer Research Campaign, the Marie Curie Foundation, as well as the HEA and the Department of Health. The Working Group has produced guidelines on sun exposure and has also initiated a Sun Awareness Week.

In the present economic climate there are many different competing demands on health resources. Although the reduction of skin cancer has been named as a government priority it still requires lobbying at all levels to ensure that it remains high on the healthcare agenda. The All Party Parliamentary Group on Skin (APPG) provides a forum where interested parties can regularly meet with MPs and peers and promote skin health at the parliamentary level. The Skin Care Campaign is an umbrella organization representing patient support groups, the HEA, the Health and Safety Executive, nursing groups, the primary care sector and the pharmaceutical industry. It too is involved with lobbying, both directly and through the APPG for a reduction in skin disease.

At the local level it is the responsibility of the public health service, working through the local service providers, to ensure that the government's health targets are met. The public health departments therefore have to set local priorities corresponding to the perceived local need. The present government has placed great importance on the development of 'partnerships' at a local level between local government, the National Health Service and the voluntary and commercial sectors. These local partnerships will be responsible for health improvement programmes. In addition it is proposed that individuals will be encouraged to play a larger role in improving their own health.

Details of two programmes

The discussion above has reviewed many aspects of educational and preventative strategies. Greater insight to the way in which these work can be gained from looking in more detail at two programmes. The first is a closer study of the Australian experience. The second is a project in North Derbyshire in which health visitors were specially trained to facilitate the development and implementation of sun safety policies in nurseries and playgroups.

Each school used the framework to create their own sun safety policy. It was endorsed by health visitors, North Derbyshire Community Health Care Services Trust and the North Derbyshire Health Promotion Services.

The Australian approach to prevention and education

'Australia is the cancer capital of the world, with 2 out of every 3 Australians developing skin cancer in their lifetime.'[16] Every year some 27 000 Australians have some form of skin cancer removed and over 1200 die from the disease, but in the last decade there has been an 11% decrease in the incidence of non-melanoma skin cancer in the under 50s. It appears that at last the massive public health campaign stimulated by the huge problem of skin cancer may be paying off. The 'Slip! Slop! Slap!' (slip on a shirt, slop on a sunscreen, slip on a hat) campaign was the first major public education campaign, mainly through school and mass media announcements throughout the summer, for several years. This was expanded into the large-scale comprehensive Sun Smart Campaign in 1988 in the state of Victoria.

For a population of 4.3 million, there was a substantial budget from the Victoria Health Promotion Foundation, funded by a levy on tobacco. In the first year Aus $994 000 was spent, which rose to Aus $1140 000 in the second. By 1997, the budget was still Aus $685 000. The aim of the campaign was to raise awareness, to model preventative behaviour and to present the Sun Smart Campaign as fashionable, particularly for young people. School children and their teachers had extensive teaching material supplied in an imaginative way, designed to interest rather than repel, educating children about the dangers, backed up by measures such as protective clothing, sunglasses and legionnaire style hats, planting shady trees in school playgrounds and reducing outdoor exposure between 11 am and 3 pm.

Links with labour unions and employers established guidelines for workers' sun protection. Cheap sunscreens were made available in large quantities and there was wide publicity about sunburn factors and ozone depletion. Because the campaigns were well funded, imaginative means of assessing their value were developed. For example, throughout the summer on a Monday evening, telephone surveys were conducted, people were interviewed about their sun exposure over the weekend, the amount of skin involved, clothing, hat and sunscreen worn and any sunburn suffered. The results suggested that a significant reduction in exposure to the risk of melanoma can be achieved in a relatively short time, with sunburn dropping from 11% to 7%, hat wearing increasing from 19% to 29% and sunscreen use from 12% to 21%. Men consistently protected themselves more than women. Adolescents and young people burnt themselves more and their behaviour has usually been particularly difficult to influence, perhaps on the basis of 'it will never happen to me' and the peer group rejection of authority.

One concern about educating people to check themselves for skin cancer is the possibility of causing needless alarm and worry. Not only may some individuals be unnecessarily anxious but it may divert attention from dangerous lesions to larger numbers of benign lesions. This could swamp the medical services, increasing the number of biopsies at enormous cost, without increasing the detection rate of melanomas. There is some evidence that this has happened.[17]

Health visitors in preschool establishments[18]

This project involved training health visitors to facilitate the development and implementation of sun safety policies in nurseries and playgroups within the boundaries of North Derbyshire Health Authority. An initial postal screening survey was conducted of all providers of preschool care or education to determine the extent to which their policies and practices were consistent with ideal sun safety practice. Those which did not have a written policy were invited to participate and be assigned randomly to either an intervention group or a control group. After training in the development and implementation of sun safety policies health visitors were matched to a local playgroup/nursery where they made three visits over a 4 month period. The outcome measures of the study were

- the number of written policies in the intervention group compared with the control group,
- the adequacy of the policy and its implementation using a 20 point scoring system and observation of the number of hats and protective clothing being worn by children and staff on a sunny day,
- knowledge and attitude questionnaire completed by nursery heads, playgroup leaders and health visitors.

Nearly 90% of playgroups and nurseries in the intervention group had developed or improved their sun safety policy whereas none in the control group had done so. One primary school had a particularly well-thought-out policy which appealed to children, parents and teachers alike. Their written policy was as follows.

The Shirebrook Model Village Primary School Sun Safety Policy

Sun Safety Policy

At Model Village Nursery we want to be sure that all children and staff are protected from skin damage caused by the harmful ultraviolet rays in the sun. We aim to do this by

- Following a structured programme of activities in all 6 areas of learning based on the theme of summer sun.
- Educating the children in what they should do to protect their skin and begin to take responsibility for their own safety.
- Encouraging children to wear clothes that provide good sun protection e.g. T shirts, sun hats, available in school for all to use.
- Scheduling outdoor activities to shaded areas during the hours 11 am–3 pm.
- Encouraging the children to use outside shady areas at all times when possible.
- Working towards increasing the amount of shade by introducing trees, thereby providing adequate shade for all those who choose to play outside.
- Encouraging staff and parents to act as good role models by practising sun safety.
- Regular reminders about sun safety through newsletters, posters and pupil activities.
- Inviting the Health Visitor to advise on Sun Safety.
- Making sure our policy is working by regularly assessing our curriculum and shade provision and reviewing the sun protection behaviour of pupils, parents and staff.

References

1. World Health Organization (1978) *Alma-Ata 1978: Primary Health Care* (WHO: Geneva).

2. UK Secretary of State for Health (1992) *The Health of the Nation* (HMSO: London).

3. Department of Health (1999) *Saving Lives: Our Healthier Nation* (TSO: London).

4. Gallagher RP, Hill GB et al (1995) Sunlight exposure, pigmentation factors and risk of non-melanoma skin cancer, II squamous cell carcinoma, *Arch Dermatol* **131**:164–9.

5. Elwood JM, Gallagher RP et al (1985) Cutaneous melanoma in relation to intermittent and constant sun exposure: The Western Canada Melanoma Study, *Int J Cancer* **35**:427–33.

6. Gallagher RP, Hill GB et al (1995) Sunlight exposure, pigmentation factors and risk of nonmelanoma skin cancer, I basal cell carcinoma, *Arch Dermatol* **131**:157–63.

7. Hill D, White V et al (1992) Melanoma prevention, behavioural and non-behavioural factors in sunburn among an Australian urban population, *Prev Med* **21**:654–69.

8. Thompson SC, Jolly D, Marks R (1993) Reduction of solar keratoses by regular sunscreen use, *N Engl J Med* **329**:1147–51.

9. Autier P, Dore JF et al (1995) Melanoma and use of sunscreens: an EORTC case-control study in Germany, Belgium and France, *Int J Cancer* **61**:749–55.

10. Welsh D, Diffey B (1981) Protection against solar actinic radiation afforded by common clothing fabrics, *Clin Exp Dermatol* **6**:577–82.

11. Wright A, Hart G, Kernohan L (1997) Dangers of sunbeds are greater in the commercial sector, *BMJ* **314**:1280–1.

12. Wilson and Junger (1968) Principles and practice of screening for disease, WHO Public Health Paper, p. 34.

13. Molina M, Rowland FS (1974) Stratospheric sink for chlorofluoromethanes, chlorine atom catalyzed destruction of ozone, *Nature* **249**:810–12.

14. Borland R, Hill D, Noy S (1990) Being 'sunsmart'; change in the community awareness and reported behaviour following a primary prevention programme for skin cancer, *Control Behav Change* **7**:126–35.

15. Smith J, Whatley P et al (1998) Improving survival of melanoma patients in Europe since 1978, *Eur J Cancer* **34**:2197–203.

16. Anti-cancer council of Victoria (1997) Annual review web site, WWW.accv.org.au.

17. Borland R, Marks R, Gibbs A et al (1995) Health effects of type of information in health education brochures upon performance on an experimental melanoma detection task. *Ed Res* **10**:191–8.

18. Syson-Nibbs LJ (submitted) Can health visitor intervention change sun safety policy and practice in preschool establishments: a randomised controlled trial, M Phil thesis submitted to Sheffield University.

Bibliography

Marks R (1999) Two decades of the public health approach to skin cancer control in Australia: why, how and where are we now? *Austr J Dermatol* **40**:1–5.

11 Psychosocial and personality factors

Introduction

This chapter is particularly relevant for patients with melanoma rather than the nonmelanoma skin cancers. The relationship between the diagnosis and course of cancer and personality types has been studied extensively. This chapter deals initially with psychological factors and prognosis. Does cancer occur more often in some personality types and do people who cope well have a better prognosis? There is relatively little literature on skin cancer and that which has been examined is on melanoma. The next part deals with psychosocial aftercare. It is thought that individuals benefit from the sense of being cared for through emotional support, information and instrumental support. These benefits may derive from psychoimmunological pathways, improving the individual's ability to cope and finally from lifestyle changes which allow them to adhere to therapy or utilize other services more readily.

Psychological factors in prognosis

It is often asked whether there is a cancer personality. The type A personality is associated with coronary-prone individuals. The theory that cancer is more likely to develop in certain types of personality is an old one. The two most frequently observed characteristics are suppression of emotion and inability to cope with interpersonal stress. Some prospective studies support the theory and if there is a causal link, it is assumed to be that hormonal and other changes result from stress in this group and that they lead to immunological deficiency that permits malignant cells to survive. Indeed stress is known to be associated with decreased natural killer cell activity, high cortisol levels, lower mucosal immunoglobulin A levels and other markers of immune status.

The next question is whether after the diagnosis of cancer the prognosis is affected by personality. Some studies have looked at psychological measures and disease progression at presentation. There is evidence that patients with the thicker malignant melanoma tumours tend to be passive and appeasing personalities. This link between poor prognosis and personality could either be via the immune system or may equally reflect a tendency for this group to seek attention too late.

The more difficult area is whether psychotherapeutic intervention could influence outcome in malignant disease and at present it can only be said that there are conflicting reports.

Psychosocial problems

There is no doubt that the diagnosis of any serious cancer is followed by degrees of psychological, psychiatric, social, occupational and sexual dysfunction for patients and their families. It rests with doctors to understand that their patients will have these problems and that being sensitive to their needs plays an important part in helping to improve their quality of life.

Uncertainty

Not knowing is a psychologically damaging experience. In many cancers there is a period of extreme concern for the patient whilst awaiting diagnostic tests. During this time the thought of cancer is predominant but uncertain. There is perversely a sense of relief when the facts are out in the open. Once a melanoma has been excised there is often only a small scar and the patient will tend to minimalize their condition. It is important that the doctor has a frank discussion about the prognosis, not to jolt the patient out of his illusion, but so that whatever the outcome, they do not lose the open and trusting relationship which would be so important in the event of metastatic disease. Melanoma is unusual among malignancies because there are some relatively good prognostic indicators. This does not mean that doctors should try and predict how long an individual will survive, but it does give a useful framework for discussion: indeed patients usually only ever ask for very rough figures such as weeks or years. Many patients like to know a timescale so that they can deal with unfinished business.

Guilt

There is a causal relationship between sun exposure and skin cancer. Patients often feel guilty that they have exposed themselves to sufficient ultraviolet light to bring this upon themselves. In addition they often wonder why they rather than somebody else who may have had even more ultraviolet exposure are victim to the disease. This can lead to further guilt, which may take strange turns as they imagine all sorts of wrong doings and that they have brought it upon themselves. Nor does guilt stop there. Often people hear that personality traits can mark people out for cancer and that prognosis may be equally effected. Also that other people combat cancer by adhering to various dietary and lifestyle changes. Inability to change their personality or to effectively alter their lifestyle can lead to feelings of helplessness and ineptitude.

Other specific fears

Often the mention of the word cancer puts people in fear of their life. For most skin tumours it is possible to allay that fear but for others the subject of death must be discussed. The fear may be of pain and loss of dignity. The extent of surgery is important because of cosmetic considerations. Large or depressed scars with skin grafts or even more mutilating surgery including amputation loom large in the patient's mind and are inseparable as body image problems from their perception of the cancer status. Most people have heard of chemotherapy and know that it can cause numerous side-effects including hair loss, nausea, vomiting and fatigue. This all adds to their fear of the future.

Psychiatric morbidity

Nearly all patients at some stage will have periods of anxiety, depression, social and sexual dysfunction. Some will go on to have persistent symptoms and studies have revealed how severe yet unrecognized the symptoms can be. Doctors have not been well trained in psychosocial aspects of disease and often rely on patients to volunteer information about depressive symptoms. Some doctors do not even believe that they should be involved with this aspect of care. Unfortunately, patients can readily detect that their tentative mention of some psychosocial aspect is met with distancing tactics from the doctor and this diminishes the strength and benefits of the relationship.

Psychological aftercare

Emotional support

Emotional support appears to be the most valuable to individuals. In one study the majority of patients defined emotional support as the most helpful followed by information support and lastly transportation support. Patients who are likely to cope badly and who may need a lot of support include those who have

- a pessimistic attitude to life,
- a psychiatric history,
- a history of alcohol or drug abuse,
- natural antagonism towards health professionals,
- a rigid lifestyle,
- low socio-economic status,
- multiple obligations.

Family support

Family are of course closest to hand for support. It is however not only the patient who feels the threat to continuity because all members fear the break-up of the family as they know it. Sometimes this may lead to family members discouraging openness and frank discussion and minimalizing the threat. There may need to be role adjustment, changes in responsibility and eventually care given to someone who previously required none. These events may cause considerable stress. Initially, the response may be a rush of activity, information gathering and false optimism. However, as the disease progresses dependence and disability increase. The inevitability of the process dawns on everyone and the emotional resources may become drained leading to a need for some support from outside the family.

Outside the family

There are many individuals and groups who can help in this area including friends, workmates and neighbours. The support may develop naturally or the patient may seek out a more formal or structured group, for example, a self-help group or support group. Cancer BACUP is a national organization that can be contacted by telephone or on the Internet. They have literature with titles such as 'Understanding malignant melanoma', 'Who can ever understand?' and 'What do I tell the children?' Their e-mail address is www.cancerbacup.org.uk and telephone number is 0800 181199. They can also put patients or their carers into contact with local people with similar problems. The need for an empathic understanding is paramount. There must be both acknowledgement of the cancer with all its ramifications and a continual relationship as individuals so that a cancer stigma does not develop. Nonempathic supporters may simply try to look on the bright side or involve the patient in activities in a way which denies acceptance of their valid difficulties. Often someone who has been through the same experience with the diagnosis of cancer will find it easier to relate in a supportive and nonthreatening way.

Medical team

The potential role of the medical team should not be underestimated. Making a diagnosis and carrying out the treatment plan is only the beginning of the story for the patient but many health professionals feel that they have almost completed their part. Not only do they have an ongoing medical role, but they are also seen as an important source of emotional support by patients. The perceived expertise and empathic understanding of a good health professional is a powerful combination and enables them to give instruction and advice which most patients find easy to accept. The team is also in a good position to look out for increasing psychological distress and to direct the patient for support as necessary. In a recent study melanoma patients were assessed for psychosocial distress, coping strategies and interest in receiving psychosocial support. Of these, 30% experienced moderate and 14% severe distress: in the latter group 83% wanted psychosocial support from their oncologist or dermatologist, but only 50% wanted to see a psychotherapist. Patients with a poor prognosis who had poor social networks and the depressive coping style showed interest in receiving support from a psychotherapist. Clearly doctors caring for melanoma patients need to be able to communicate supportively and identify those who are not adjusting to their illness.

Information support

At the time of diagnosis it is difficult for the patient to retain information and although there may be a relative or friend present, it is not the best time to go into detail regarding prognosis, treatment protocols and so on. At subsequent visits and as time goes on there will be differing needs for further information. Some individuals ask little and even resist a detailed explanation of their condition. Others want precise statistical information relating to their tumour.

By the time a patient has come to a follow-up visit and is seeking more information, they may have gleaned a considerable knowledge base of their own, but it is usually not seen in a proper perspective. The sources of information are variable such as a fellow sufferer, a self-help group, a library, a magazine, a television programme and of course most recently the Internet. It is possible to connect with cancer institutions and there are medically orientated on-line services. It may be helpful to suggest these resources to those who have not considered them, but it is also useful to ask to which sources patients have access so that the doctor knows what sort of information the patient is being guided by. For instance the approach to chemotherapy for melanoma may be different in Singapore or mainland Europe and it would be important to explain why the same approach was not used in the UK.

Instrumental support

As the individual becomes more dependent, the need for practical help increases. The ability of family to provide this may diminish through a long illness so that formal systems need to be utilized. In the UK healthcare is free at the point of its provision. This means that all costs for inpatient and outpatient care are provided by the National Health Service. Anticancer drugs are similarly available. Other prescriptions and certain equipment may bear a standard charge. The situation in other countries differs widely and without full health insurance cover, some individuals are put under a severe financial burden and may need to borrow money to pay for their care. Loss of income is accompanied by some areas of increased expenditure such as transportation, parking and childcare. Transportation is often a problem even for those with their own car because general debility and the effects of some of the medications can make driving unsafe. Increasingly cancer care is to be provided in cancer centres which are few and far between and will necessitate even longer journeys. It has been shown that for people with limited financial means the provision of transport leads to an increased number keeping their medical appointments.

Medical equipment comprises such items as wheelchairs, wheelchair ramps, bath hoists and dressings. Agencies including social services, district nursing services and primary healthcare teams arrange for these items to be delivered to the home.

In addition to the statutory bodies involved in the provision of instrumental support, there are numerous voluntary and charitable bodies whose activities enhance the quality of life and care of cancer patients. It is usually the hospital team or social services personnel who are able to advise on the appropriate contacts in the charity framework.

Appendix I
Guidelines for management of Bowen's disease

NH Cox, DJ Eedy and CA Morton

Summary

These guidelines for management of Bowen's disease have been prepared for dermatologists on behalf of the British Association of Dermatologists. They present evidence-based guidance for treatment, with identification of the strength of evidence available at the time of preparation of the guidelines, and a brief overview of epidemiological aspects, diagnosis and investigation.

Definition and introduction to the guideline

Bowen's disease (BD) is a form of intraepidermal (in situ) squamous cell carcinoma (SCC), originally described in 1912.[1] It is usually persistent and progressive, with a small potential for invasive malignancy, although spontaneous partial regression may occur. Its epidemiology, predisposing factors, disease associations and risk of malignancy are all pertinent to patient management and are discussed in addition to the local treatment options for the disease itself.

Histology

The epidermis is replaced by abnormal keratinocytes with disordered maturation and loss of polarity. Large and atypical mitotic figures are characteristic. Similar changes extend deeply into the pilosebaceous unit and may replace the infundibulum, external root sheath and sebaceous gland[2] (a feature which may explain recurrences after superficial forms of therapy). DNA-ploidy studies also support the malignant nature of BD, although DNA malignancy grades are lower than for SCC.[3] Large cell acanthoma may be a rare cytologic variant of BD.[4]

Clinical description, demographics and variants

Typical BD presents as a gradually enlarging well demarcated erythematous plaque with an irregular border and surface crusting or scaling.[5] Symptoms are minor in the absence of ulceration. BD may occur at any age in adults but is rare before the age of 30 years; most patients are aged over 60.[5–12] In the U.K., the peak age group is the seventh decade.[6,7] Lesions are usually solitary but are multiple in 10–20% of patients.[6–10] Any site may be affected, although involvement of palms[13,14] or soles is uncommon. In the U.K., BD occurs predominantly in women (70–85% of cases),[6,7] and about three-quarters of patients have lesions on the lower leg (60–85%).[6,7]

Specific sites which deserve mention due to the potential for diagnostic confusion include perianal[15–17] and subungual BD.[18–20] Pigmented BD is an uncommon variant, occurring in 1·7% of cases in one series,[21] and is particularly likely at flexural, perianal or subungual sites. Verrucous BD is important as it is likely to raise suspicion of invasive carcinoma.

Genital lesions which have the histology of BD include erythroplasia of Queyrat and Bowenoid papulosis.[22–26] Erythroplasia of Queyrat (penile intraepithelial neoplasia) occurs on the glans penis and under the prepuce, virtually always in uncircumcised men. Comments on vulval BD in these guidelines are drawn from references written over several years, which may have included both lesions morphologically similar to BD at other body sites and other dysplastic lesions which would be classified as vulval intraepithelial neoplasia (VIN) according to current terminology. Reference to original data sources and current vulval disease literature is recommended if treating VIN. Bowenoid papulosis is a different disorder with a viral aetiology, slight female predominance and benign behaviour in most cases, but it may cause extensive multiple lesions.

Rarely, BD may affect other mucosal surfaces such as oral mucosa and the conjunctiva or cornea;[27] these are not discussed further.

Aetiology

Solar

The age group and body site distribution of BD (head and neck, female lower leg) are suggestive of a relationship with chronic solar damage.[4,9,11] As with other skin cancers, BD is rare in individuals with black skin in whom it predominantly affects non-exposed sites.[28] BD has been reported in patients having psoralen ultraviolet A treatment.[29–31]

Arsenic

Several studies have identified an association between BD and previous arsenic exposure.[32–35] In one large survey, about 50% of arsenical cancers were BD,[32,33] although another study reported that multiple basal cell carcinomas were the commonest arsenical tumour and were more frequent than multiple or solitary BD.[34] There is typically a time lag of over 10 years (often several decades) between exposure and development of BD.

Immunosuppression

There are small numbers of reported cases of BD associated with congenital or acquired immunosuppression, including patients with AIDS. BD is probably not uncommon in transplant patients having therapeutic immunosuppression, but is not separately identified in all studies.

Viral

A number of viral agents have been implicated in the aetiology of BD. The most extensively investigated have been human papilloma viruses (HPV), especially HPV16, which have been detected in up to 20–30% of anogenital lesions,[36,37] although some large studies have reported much lower[38] or negative[39] results. Human herpesvirus type 8 has been reported in up to two-thirds of BD lesions[40,41] but was not found in another study.[42]

Other aetiological agents and pre-existing lesions Therapeutic and other ionizing radiation has been reported to cause BD, as have various forms of skin injury or chronic dermatoses (such as lupus vulgaris or chronic lupus erythematosus[12]).

There are several cases of BD arising in seborrhoeic keratoses[43] and it has also been reported in porokeratoses (disseminated, Mibelli and linear types) and in a Becker's naevus.

Association with internal malignancy

The apparent relationship between BD and internal malignancy was reported in 1959[44] and several studies subsequently supported this association.[6,45–48] Multiple lesions of BD have been associated with higher risk but not confirmed in a U.K. population.[6] However, some studies found no significant association with internal malignancy for BD overall,[49] or for BD at specific sites such as perianal BD.[50] A critical analysis review of the existing studies in 1987 concluded that there were many methodological concerns,[51] and a subsequent meta-analysis of 12 studies in 1989 indicated that there was no significant association.[52] The overall conclusion from larger studies and meta-analysis is therefore that routine investigation for internal malignancy in patients with BD is not justified (strength of evidence, E).

Association with other skin malignancy

In studies which have examined this association, about 30–50% of subjects had other previous or subsequent skin malignancies (mainly basal cell carcinoma).[8,9] The standardized incidence ratio for subsequent non-melanoma skin cancer was 4·3 in a recent study.[53]

Risk of progression to squamous cell carcinoma

Although risk of progression to invasive SCC of up to 20% has been suggested, most studies suggest a risk of invasive carcinoma of about 3%.[46,54] Of these, one-third may metastasize.[54] However, both of these figures are drawn from retrospective case series. When invasion occurs it may have sebaceous or eccrine differentiation.[56,57] The degree of aneuploidy in BD has been proposed as a factor to predict risk of invasive carcinoma,[58] but other authors feel that aneuploidy occurs in all BD and is unlikely to have prognostic significance.[59]

The risk of invasion for genital BD or erythroplasia of Queyrat, in the region of 10%,[7,22,23] is greater than for typical sites of BD. In Bowenoid papulosis invasion is extremely rare,[23] but cervical intraepithelial carcinoma (CIN) occurs in 60–90% of affected females or in female sex partners of affected men,[60] and oral papillomas and tumours have been reported in association with HPV16-positive Bowenoid papulosis. Perianal BD also has higher risk of invasion, recurrence, and an association with cervical and vulvar dysplasia.[16,17] The risk of invasive carcinoma may also be higher for BD on the neck compared with other sites (10% in one study,[8] compared with an overall risk for all sites of 4% in the same study population).

Investigation and diagnosis

Diagnosis is primarily on the basis of clinical features. Histological confirmation is required for cases with diagnostic doubt, or where there is suspicion of invasive malignancy. Biopsy is probably not required for all small lesions diagnosed by specialists; clinicopathological correlation was good in one study[7] but this has not been extensively investigated.

Treatment

Evaluation of treatment studies of BD is difficult due to potential selection bias to specific forms of treatment. Similarly, healing and success rate may vary with body site. Virtually all authors use visible rather than histological assessment to determine the end-point of clearance. Even for the same treatment modality, there is difficulty in directly comparing studies due to different lesion sites, sizes of lesions and use of different types of equipment and treatment regimens.

No treatment

In some patients with slowly progressive thin lesions, especially on the elderly lower leg where healing is poor, there is an argument for observation rather than intervention.

5-Fluorouracil (strength of evidence B, II–iii [Appendix])

5-Fluorouracil has been used topically for treatment of BD in several studies.[61–66] Most of these are open trials or small case series. It is usually applied once or twice daily as a 5% cream for a variable period of time (between 1 week and 2 months in most studies using this concentration) to achieve disease control, and repeated if required at intervals. Efficacy may be increased by application under occlusion,[62] and a recent study used iontophoresis to improve follicular penetration.[64] In this study,[64] only one of 26 patients had histological evidence of residual disease at 3 months after eight treatments (evidence II–iii). It has been combined with dinitrochlorobenzene (DNCB) to improve penetration, but the DNCB appeared to be the effective constituent.[65] An evaluation of different concentrations of 5FU (in a propylene glycol base) used mainly a 1% strength for 4–18 weeks (most 8–12 weeks) in 41 patients, with an 8% recurrence rate; the authors suggested that at least 2·5% was required for BD at extrafacial sites.[62] As 5FU can be very irritant, less aggressive regimens have been used for disease control rather than cure. A once weekly application of 5% 5FU improved lesions in 24 of 26 patients, although long-term clearance was only achieved in a minority with this regimen.[66]

In erythroplasia of Queyrat, application of 5% cream twice daily for 4–5 weeks has been recommended,[26,67] but inflammation frequently limits this treatment regimen.[22]

None of these studies provide details of the success rate for the currently available preparation available in the U.K. (5% cream to be used once or twice daily for 3–4 weeks) as a first-line option for unselected lesions.

Cryotherapy (strength of evidence A, II–i)

The varied results reported may reflect differences between studies in equipment and regimen used. Thestrup–Pedersen et al.[8] reported a 33% failure rate in 56 patients but the regimen was not provided. The studies discussed below all used liquid nitrogen (LN_2) cryotherapy.

Plaza de Lanza and colleagues using LN_2 in 28 patients with BD[68] demonstrated that a single freeze–thaw cycle (FTC) of 30 s was as effective as 2×30 s (no failures or recurrences in either group) but more effective than 1×15 s (two failures and one recurrence). Graham and Clark[69] reported one recurrence in 30 patients treated with a single FTC of LN_2 of sufficient duration to produce a clinical thaw time of at least 90 s. Holt[70] treated 128 lesions of BD (including 20 lesions > 2 cm diameter) in 85 patients under lignocaine local anaesthesia, with the same single 30 s FTC of LN_2. There was only 1 in 128 recurrence during a minimum 1-year follow-up period, in a 2-cm lesion on the calf which was later demonstrated to have a focus of invasive cancer. Slow healing of the lower leg was noted.

Cox and Dyson[71] used LN_2 with two FTC of 20 s for 82 lesions on the lower leg in 49 patients (including 17 lesions > 2 cm diameter), and demonstrated recurrence in five patients (6%) after a minimum 1-year follow-up; one of these had a focus of invasive cancer which was not apparent in a pretreatment incisional biopsy. No anaesthesia was required, and there were no treatment-related failures of healing, but lesions of > 2 cm were treated in a staged manner at 2-month intervals.

Morton et al.[72] reported 100% clearance in 20 patients with one to three treatments of LN_2 using one FTC of 20 s on each occasion (50% success after a single treatment). There were two (10%) recurrences in the 1-year follow-up period. In this study, photodynamic therapy was more effective than cryotherapy but the FTC duration was less than in the studies detailed above; despite this, five lesions ulcerated following cryotherapy.

The combination of intermittent cryotherapy before and during 4 weeks of 5FU was used for a technically difficult ear lesion with success, but in a single case and with focal recurrences.[73]

Cryotherapy therefore appears to have a good success rate (recurrences less than 10% at 12 months) but healing may be slow for broad lesions and discomfort may limit treatment of multiple lesions.

Curettage with cautery/electrocautery (strength of evidence A, II–iii)

Veien et al. did not report any recurrences within 2 years among 33 cases of BD treated with curettage and electrocautery, compared with 36 of 508 basal cell carcinoma recurrences in the same treatment period.[75] However, recurrence rates of 20% were reported by both Thestrup-Pedersen et al.[8] (65 of 345 cases) and by Sturm[62] (four of 20 cases) with this modality, and a 73% failure rate was recorded by Graham and Helwig,[45] although these studies do not give details of the treatment regimens or equipment. Healing has recently been demonstrated to be faster after curettage than after cryotherapy with less early pain,[74] but the variable and possibly suboptimal cryotherapy in this study (some lesions treated with 2FTC of 5 s) does not permit firm conclusions regarding recurrence rates.

Excision (strength of evidence A, II–iii)

Thestrup–Pedersen et al. reported a 4·5% recurrence rate (three of 65 cases) with simple excision.[8] Graham and Helwig[45] treated 62% of 155 patients by excision only, and had a 19% recurrence rate within 5 years. The risk of recurrence after simple excision is greater at some sites, such as perianal BD (discussed later).

Mohs micrographic surgery has been used for lesions at special sites such as the penis, where tissue sparing is important, with good results in the small number of reported cases.[76]

Laser (strength of evidence B, III)

Lasers used to treat BD include CO^2, argon and Nd:YAG.[77–79] They have particularly been used to treat lesions at difficult sites such as the finger or genitalia, and CO_2 laser has also been used to treat Bowenoid papulosis. Results are generally stated to be good, but the published results are of small numbers, or are considered with other epidermal neoplasia and difficult to analyse specifically.

Photodynamic therapy (strength of evidence A, II–iii)

This modality requires the activation of a photosensitizer, usually a porphyrin deriva-tive, by visible light. Systemic photosensiti-zation was used with excellent results in early studies[80,81] but this summary refers to aminolaevulinic acid (ALA)–photodynamic therapy (PDT) (PDT using topical ALA derivatives).

Svanberg et al. reported complete response in nine of 10 cases of BD (2–5 cm diameter) treated with d-ALA and 60 J/cm² of 630 nm laser light.[82] Epithelialization was established at 3–6 weeks and there were no recurrences over 6–14 months. Cairnduff et al.[83] achieved initial clearance of 35 of 36 lesions of BD (one partial response) using 5-ALA and 125–150 J/cm² of 630 nm laser light; three cases relapsed at a median follow-up of 18 months (overall success 89%). Stables et al.[84] reported a complete clinical response in 73 of 77 lesions in 54 patients at 12 months (71 of 77 at 24 months) using ALA and either 125 J/cm² white light from a modified slide projector or 100–125 J/cm² of 630 nm laser light. The same authors have reported the successful use of ALA–PDT for broad lesions of BD in three patients[85] (each required two treatments) and for erythroplasia of Queyrat.[86]

Morton et al.[72] demonstrated clearance in 20 of 20 lesions of BD (75% with one, 25% with two treatments) using 5-ALA and 125 J/cm²   xenon   arc   irradiation (630 ± 615 nm), with no recurrences at 12 months. Varma et al. have recently used a non-laser red light source[87] to treat 38 lesions of BD, with 95% complete response after two treatments which was sustained at 12 months in 15 of 19 who were reviewed.

The currently reported overall initial clinical clearance rate for ALA–PDT is therefore 90–100%, and recurrence rate 0–11% in studies with completed 12-month follow-up. Good cosmesis and healing is likely, but avail-ability is limited.

Radiotherapy (strength of evidence B, II–iii)

A variety of radiotherapy techniques and regimens have been used to treat BD, including external beam irradiation, strontium 90, proton radiotherapy and beta-emitting radionuclides. Although Graham and Helwig reported an 88% failure rate in 12 patients,[45] complete response rates of 100% were reported in 77 lesions treated with X-irradiation by Blank and Schnyder,[88] and in 59 patients treated by Cox and Dyson.[71] In one of these studies,[88] two patients (both with genital lesions) relapsed at 8 and 16 months. The patients reported by Cox and Dyson all had lower leg lesions, and poor healing (which was related to age, diameter of field and radiotherapy dose) was a feature in 12 of 59 (20%). Thus the high cure rate may be offset by impaired healing.

Other treatments

The combination of isotretinoin and interferon alpha has been used in one patient with multiple lesions of BD (over 50 plaques) and all except two cleared after 3 months of treatment with sustained remission at 15 months.[89] Etretinate and interferon gamma have both also been used for treatment of Bowenoid papulosis.

Site-specific treatment

Digits

Excision has usually been recommended at digital/subungual sites.[18,19] A study of seven cases recommended Mohs surgery for optimal tissue sparing.[19] CO_2 laser may also be useful, with 80% cure in a series of five patients.[78]

Genital

Erythroplasia of Queyrat has higher risks of invasion compared with ordinary BD, and treatment may need to be more aggressive. Mohs surgery has been advised for tissue sparing, and CO_2 laser for good healing. However, radiotherapy, 5FU, PDT[86] and cryotherapy[90] are all potentially useful.

Bowenoid papulosis has very low risk, and treatment is dictated by the multiplicity of lesions; the risk of CIN in women is important.

Perianal Bowen's disease

Treatment is usually surgical or with radiotherapy. Wide local excision is usually adequate[15–17] but has a recurrence rate of 10–30%; the rate after simple excision may be over 50%.[17] In one study of 47 cases, the recurrence rate after CO_2 laser was 80% (four of five cases) but after wide excision was 23% (six of 26 cases).[17] A study of 57 cases of epidermoid carcinoma of the anal margin[91] suggested that radiotherapy is the treatment of choice for BD but did not specifically present any results for this disorder. PDT has been used in a small number of cases.

Treatment failures and relapses

Treatment failure may be related to indistinct margins (marginal recurrences), concern about healing and minimizing damage to normal tissues, extension of BD down follicles (a typical histological feature) and unrecognized foci of invasive tumour (usually not marginal). Attempts to identify margins more accurately using acetowhitening were reported as useful in one study of 12 lesions[92] but unreliable in another study of eight patients.[93]

Table 1
Summary of the main treatment options for Bowen's disease. The suggested strengths of the treatments listed takes into account the evidence for benefit, ease of application or time required for the procedure, wound healing, cosmetic result and availability of the method or facilities required.

Lesion characteristics	Cryo-therapy	Curettage	Excision	Topical 5-fluorouracil	Photodynamic therapy	Radio-therapy
Small, single, good healing[a]	1	2	3	4	3	5
Large, single, good healing[a]	3	5	5	3	2	4
Multiple, good healing[a]	2	3	5	3	3	4
Small, poor healing site[a]	3	2	2	2	2	5
Large, poor healing site[a]	5	4	5	3	2	6
Facial	2	2	4	4	3	4
Digital	3	5	4	3	3	3
Perianal	6	6	1	6	7	3
Penile	3	5	4	3	3	3

[a]Refers to the clinician's perceived potential for good or poor healing at the affected site.
1, Probably treatment of choice; 2, generally good choice; 3, generally fair choice; 4, reasonable but not usually required; 5, generally poor choice;6, probably should not be used; 7, insufficient evidence available.

Summary of treatment modalities

Most of the above treatments have good success rates, but all have a risk of slow healing at the characteristic lower leg site of BD seen in the U.K. The potential benefits of each treatment are offset by limitations. Thus, for example: laser and PDT treatments have high cost and/or limited availability; simple excision and Mohs surgery are time-consuming and wound closure is difficult on the lower leg; cryotherapy and PDT cause discomfort; and radiotherapy has a high success rate but significant failure to heal on the lower leg. Cryotherapy and curettage are the cheapest and most available of the surgical modalities. The relative status of the available treatment options is summarized in Table 1. This takes into account the evidence for benefit, ease of application and time required for the technique, wound healing, cosmetic result and availability of the method or facilities required.

Follow-up

Required duration of follow-up is uncertain, in part because many studies have used 12-month follow-up periods and clinical assessment for the detection of recurrences. In a series of various epidermal tumours treated with cryotherapy, Holt recommended a 2-year follow-up period on the basis that only one recurrence was after 18 months; however, this series included several different tumour types, and the one BD recurrence was at 6 months.[70] Most recurrences after PDT have been detected within 2 years. In a series of 19 patients with perianal BD[16] the recurrence rate increased from 16% at 1 year to 31% at 5 years; longer follow-up may therefore be appropriate for BD at less common and less visible sites, or where HPV infection is likely to have been relevant. However, in determining follow-up it is not simply the index lesion which is relevant, as a significant proportion of patients have multiple lesions or other epidermal neoplasia at presentation or subsequently.

In uncomplicated cases of solitary BD we suggest that review at about 3 months to confirm clearance and healing is prudent. The requirement for subsequent review should take into account the presence of multiple lesions, previous recurrence, other skin neoplasia, the reliability of the patient and the degree of primary care support.

Conclusions

1. There is no convincing evidence to support routine screening for internal cancer in patients with BD.
2. The risk of progression to invasive cancer is about 3%.
3. There is a significant frequency of multiple lesions and an association of BD with other skin cancers, which may reflect the predominantly solar aetiology or, in some cases, arsenic exposure.
4. Genital, and particularly perianal, BD have higher risks of invasive cancer.
5. Treatment options for BD include cryotherapy, curettage, excision, laser, photodynamic therapy and topical 5FU; all of these have recurrence rates in the order of 5–10%, and no treatment modality appears to be superior for all clinical situations.
6. Direct comparison between treatment modalities is difficult as there are few randomized clinical trials with comparable patient subgroups; other factors such as treatment-related morbidity and the costs and availability of the treatment options need to be considered.

References

1 Bowen JT. Precancerous dermatoses: a study of two cases of chronic atypical epithelial proliferation. *J Cutan Dis* 1912; **30**: 241–55.
2 Strayer DS, Santa Cruz DJ. Carcinoma in situ of the skin: a review of histopathology. *J Cutan Pathol* 1980; **7**: 244–59.
3 Bocking A, Chatelain R, Salterberg A, Hagedorn M, Gross G. Bowenoid papulosis. Classification as a low-grade in situ carcinoma of the epidermis on the basis of histomorphologic and DNA ploidy studies. *Anal Quant Cytol Histol* 1989; **11**: 419–25.
4 Sanchez Yus E, de Diego V, Urrutia S. Large cell acanthoma. A cytologic variant of Bowen's disease? *Am J Dermatopath* 1988; **10**: 197–208.
5 Lee M-M, Wick MM. Bowen's disease. *CA Cancer J Clin* 1990; **40**: 237–42.
6 Eedy DJ, Gavin AT. Thirteen-year retrospective study of Bowen's disease in Northern Ireland. *Br J Dermatol* 1987; **117**: 715–20.
7 Cox NH. Body site distribution of Bowen's disease. *Br J Dermatol* 1994; **130**: 714–16.
8 Thestrup-Pedersen K, Ravnborg L, Reymann F. Morbus Bowen. *Acta Derm Venereol (Stockh)* 1988; **68**: 236–9.
9 Reizner GT, Chuang TY, Elpern DJ, Stone JL, Farmer ER. Bowen's disease (squamous cell carcinoma in situ) in Kauai, Hawaii. A population-based incidence report. *J Am Acad Dermatol* 1994; **31**: 596–600.
10 Kovacs A, Yonemoto K, Katsuoka K, Nishiyama S, Harhai I. Bowen's disease: statistical study of a 10 year period. *J Dermatol* 1996; **23**: 267–74.
11 Kossard S, Rosen R. Cutaneous Bowen's disease. An analysis of 1001 cases according

to age, sex, and site. *J Am Acad Dermatol* 1992; **27**: 406–10.

12 Degos R, Civatte J, Letessier S. Maladie de Bowen cutanee ou muqueuse. *Ann Dermatol Syphiligr* 1976; **103**: 5–14.

13 Binet O, Beltzer-Garelli E, Elbaz JS, Aron-Brunetiere R. Bowen's disease and squamous cell carcinoma of the palm. *Dermatologica* 1980; **161**: 136–9.

14 Gonzalez-Perez R, Gardeazabal J, Eizaguirre X, Diaz-Perez JL. Metastatic squamous cell carcinoma arising in Bowen's disease of the palm. *J Am Acad Dermatol* 1997; **36**: 635–6.

15 Beck DE, Fazio VW, Jagelman DG, Lavery IC. Perianal Bowen's disease. *Dis Colon Rectum* 1988; **31**: 419–22.

16 Sarmiento JM, Wolff BG, Burgart LJ, Frizelle FA, Ilstrup DM. Perianal Bowen's disease: associated tumors, human papillomavirus, surgery, and other controversies. *Dis Colon Rectum* 1997; **40**: 912–18.

17 Marchesa P, Fazio VW, Oliart S, Goldblum JR, Lavery IC. Perianal Bowen's disease: a clinicopathological study of 47 patients. *Dis Colon Rectum* 1997; **40**: 1286–93.

18 Baran R, Dupre A, Sayag J, Letessier S, Robins P, Bureau H. Bowen disease of the nail apparatus. *Ann Dermatol Venereol* 1979; **106**: 227–33.

19 Sau P, McMarlin SL, Sperling LC, Katz R. Bowen's disease of the nail bed and periungual area. A clinicopathologic analysis of seven cases. *Arch Dermatol* 1994; **130**: 204–9.

20 Goodman G, Mason G, O'Brien T. Polydactylous Bowen's disease of the nail bed. *Austral J Dermatol* 1995; **36**: 164–5.

21 Ragi G, Turner MS, Klein LE, Stoll HL. Pigmented Bowen's disease and review of 420 Bowen's disease lesions. *J Dermatol Surg Oncol* 1988; **14**: 765–9.

22 Mikhail GR. Cancers, precancers, and pseudocancers on the male genitalia. *J Dermatol Surg Oncol* 1980; **6**: 1027–35.

23 Patterson JW, Kao GF, Graham JH, Helwig EB. Bowenoid papulosis. A clinicopathologic study with ultrastructural observations. *Cancer* 1986; **57**: 823–36.

24 Gerber GS. Carcinoma in situ of the penis. *J Urol* 1994; **151**: 829–33.

25 Schwartz RA, Janniger CK. Bowenoid papulosis. *J Am Acad Dermatol* 1991; **24**: 261–4.

26 Goette K. Review of erythroplasia of Queyrat and its treatment. *Urol* 1976; **8**: 311–15.

27 Sanders N, Bedotto C. Recurrent carcinoma in situ of the conjunctiva and cornea (Bowen's disease). *Am J Ophthalmol* 1972; **74**: 688–93.

28 Mora RG, Perniciaro C, Lee B. Cancer of the skin in blacks. III. A review of nineteen black patients with Bowen's disease. *J Am Acad Dermatol* 1984; **11**: 557–62.

29 Hofmann C, Plewig G, Braun-Falco O. Bowenoid lesions, Bowen's disease and keratoacanthomas in long-term PUVA-treated patients. *Br J Dermatol* 1979; **101**: 685–92.

30 Reshad H, Challoner F, Pollock DJ, Baker H. Cutaneous carcinoma in psoriatic patients treated with PUVA. *Br J Dermatol* 1984; **110**: 299–305.

31 McKenna KE, Paterson CC, Handley J, McGinn S, Allen G. Cutaneous neoplasia following PUVA therapy for psoriasis. *Br J Dermatol* 1996; **134**: 639–42.

32 Yeh S, How SW, Lin CS. Arsenical cancer of the skin. Histologic study with special reference to Bowen's disease. *Cancer* 1968; **21**: 312–39.

33 Yeh S. Skin cancer in chronic arsenicism. *Hum Pathol* 1967; **4**: 469–85.

34 Fiertz U. Catamnestic investigations of the side effects of therapy of skin diseases with inorganic arsenic. *Dermatologica* 1965; **131**: 41–58.

35 Shannon RL, Strayer DS. Arsenic-induced skin toxicity. *Hum Toxicol* 1989; **8**: 99–104.

36 Kettler AH, Rutledge M, Tschen JA, Buffone G. Detection of human papillomavirus in nongenital Bowen's disease by in situ DNA hybridization. *Arch Dermatol* 1990; **126**: 777–81.

37 Collina G, Rossi E, Betelli S et al. Detection of human papillomavirus in extragenital Bowen's disease using in situ hybridization

and polymerase chain reaction. *Am J Dermatopath* 1995; **17**: 236–41.

38 Kawashima M, Favre M, Obalek S, Jablonska S, Orth G. Premalignant lesions and cancers of the skin in the general population: evaluation of the role of human papillomaviruses. *J Invest Dermatol* 1990; **95**: 537–42.

39 Lu S, Syrjanen K, Havu VK, Syrjanen S. Failure to demonstrate human papillomavirus (HPV) involvement in Bowen's disease of the skin. *Arch Dermatol Res* 1996; **289**: 40–5.

40 Inagi R, Kosuge H, Nishimoto S, Yoshikawa K, Yamanishi K. Kaposi's sarcoma-associated herpesvirus (KSHV) sequences in premalignant and malignant skin tumors. *Arch Virol* 1996; **141**: 2217–23.

41 Nishimoto S, Inagi R, Yamanishi K, Hosokawa K, Kakibuchi M, Yoshikawa K. Prevalence of human herpesvirus-8 in skin lesions. *Br J Dermatol* 1997; **137**: 179–84.

42 Mitsuishi T, Sata T, Matsukura T, Kawashima M. Human herpes-virus 8 DNA is rarely found in Bowen's disease of non-immunosuppressed patients. *Br J Dermatol* 1997; **136**: 803–4.

43 Cascajo CD, Reichel M, Sanchez JL. Malignant neoplasms associated with seborrheic keratoses. An analysis of 54 cases. *Am J Dermatopathol* 1996; **18**: 278–82.

44 Graham JH, Helwig EB. Bowen's disease and its relationship to systemic cancer. *Arch Dermatol* 1959; **80**: 133–59.

45 Graham JH, Helwig EB. Bowen's disease and its relationship to systemic cancer. *Arch Dermatol* 1961; **83**: 76–96.

46 Peterka ES, Lynch FW, Goltz RW. An association between Bowen's disease and cancer. *Arch Dermatol* 1961; **84**: 623–9.

47 Callen JP, Headington J. Bowen's and non-Bowen's squamous intraepithelial neoplasia of the skin. Relationship to internal malignancy. *Arch Dermatol* 1980; **116**: 422–6.

48 Chute CG, Chuang TY, Bergstralh EJ, Su WP. The subsequent risk of internal cancer with Bowen's disease. A population-based study. *JAMA* 1991; **266**: 816–19.

49 Reymann F, Ravnborg L, Schou G, Engholm G, Osterlind A, Thestrup-Pedersen K. Bowen's disease and internal malignant diseases: a study 581 patients. *Arch Dermatol* 1988; **124**: 677–9.

50 Marfing TE, Abel ME, Gallagher DM. Perianal Bowen's disease and associated malignancies. Results of a survey. *Dis Colon Rectum* 1987; **30**: 782–5.

51 Arbesmann H, Ransohoff DF. Is Bowen's disease a predictor for the development of internal malignancy? A methodological critique of the literature. *JAMA* 1987; **257**: 516–18.

52 Lycka BAS. Bowen's disease and internal malignancy. A meta-analysis. *Int J Dermatol* 1989; **28**: 531–3.

53 Jaeger AB, Gramkow A, Hjalgrim H et al. Bowen disease and risk of subsequent malignant neoplasms. A population-based cohort study of 1147 patients *Arch Dermatol* 1999; **135**: 790–793.

54 Kao GF. Carcinoma arising in Bowen's disease. *Arch Dermatol* 1986; **122**: 1124–6.

55 Stout AP. Malignant manifestations of Bowen's disease. *NY J Med* 1939; **39**: 801–9.

56 Jacobs DM, Sandles LG, Leboit PE. Sebaceous carcinoma arising from Bowen's disease of the vulva. *Arch Dermatol* 1986; **122**: 1191–3.

57 Saida T, Okabe Y, Uhara H. Bowen's disease with invasive carcinoma showing sweat gland differentiation. *J Cutan Pathol* 1989; **16**: 222–6.

58 Biesterfeld S, Pennings K, Grussendorf-Conen EI, Bocking A. Aneuploidy in actinic keratosis and Bowen's disease–increased risk for invasive squamous cell carcinoma? *Br J Dermatol* 1995; **133**: 557–60.

59 Newton JA, Camplejohn RS, McGibbon DH. Aneuploidy in Bowen's disease. *Br J Dermatol* 1986; **114**: 691–4.

60 Obalek S, Jablonska S, Beaudenon S, Walczak L, Orth G. Bowenoid papulosis of the male and female genitalia: risk of cervical neoplasia. *J Am Acad Dermatol* 1986; **14**: 433–44.

61 Tolia BM, Castro VL, Mouded IM, Newman

HR. Bowen's disease of shaft of penis. Successful treatment with 5-fluorouracil. *Urology* 1976; **7**: 617–19.

62 Sturm HM. Bowen's disease and 5-fluorouracil. *J Am Acad Dermatol* 1979; **16**: 513–22.

63 Fulton JE Jr, Carter DM, Hurley HJ. Treatment of Bowen's disease with topical 5-fluorouracil under occlusion. *Arch Dermatol* 1968; **97**: 178–80.

64 Welch ML, Grabski WJ, McCollough ML et al. 5-fluorouracil iontophoretic therapy for Bowen's disease;. *J Am Acad Dermatol* 1997; **36**: 956–8.

65 Raaf JH, Krown SE, Pinsky CM et al. Treatment of Bowen's disease with topical dinitrochlorobenzene and 5-fluorouracil. *Cancer* 1967; **37**: 1633–42.

66 Stone N, Burge S. Bowen's disease of the leg treated with weekly pulses of 5% fluorouracil cream. *Br J Dermatol* 1999; **140**: 987–8.

67 Jansen GT, Dillaha CJ, Honeycutt WM. Bowenoid conditions of the skin: treatment with topical 5-fluorouracil. *Southern Med J* 1967; **60**: 185–8.

68 Plaza Lanza M, Ralphs I, Dawber RPR. Cryosurgery for Bowen's disease of the skin. *Br J Dermatol* 1980; **103** (**Suppl. 18**): 14.

69 Graham GF, Clark LC. Statistical update in cryosurgery for cancers of the skin. In: Cryosurgery for Skin Cancers and Cutaneous Disorders (Zacarian S, ed.). St Louis: Mosby, 1985; 298–305.

70 Holt PJ. Cryotherapy for skin cancer: results over a 5-year period using liquid nitrogen spray cryosurgery. *Br J Dermatol* 1988; **119**: 231–40.

71 Cox NH, Dyson P. Wound healing on the lower leg after radiotherapy or cryotherapy of Bowen's disease and other malignant skin lesions. *Br J Dermatol* 1995; **133**: 60–5.

72 Morton CA, Whitehurst C, Moseley H, McColl JH, Moore JV, Mackie RM. Comparison of photodynamic therapy with cryotherapy in the treatment of Bowen's disease. *Br J Dermatol* 1995; **135**: 766–71.

73 Heising RA. Treatment of Bowen's disease of the ear by the combined use of cryosurgery and topical 5-fluorouracil. *Cutis* 1979; **24**: 271–5.

74 Ahmed I, Berth-Jones J, Charles-Holmes S, Ilchyshyn A. Comparison of cryotherapy versus curretage in the treatment of Bowen's disease. *Br J. Dermatol* 1999; **141** (**Suppl. 55**): 31.

75 Veien SK, Veien NK, Hattel T, Laurberg G. Results of treatment of non-melanoma skin cancer in a dermatologic practice. A prospective study. *Ugeskrift Laeger* 1996; **158**: 7213–5.

76 Moritz DL, Lynch WS. Extensive Bowen's disease of the penile shaft treated with fresh tissue Mohs micrographic surgery in two separate operations. *J Dermatol Surg Oncol* 1991; **17**: 374–8.

77 Boynton KK, Bjorkman DJ. Argon laser therapy for perianal Bowen's disease: a case report. *Lasers Surg Med* 1991; **11**: 385–7.

78 Gordon KB, Garden JM, Robinson JK. Bowen's disease of the distal digit. Outcome of treatment with carbon dioxide laser vaporization. *Dermatol Surg* 1996; **22**: 723–8.

79 Landthaler M, Haina D, Brunner R et al. Laser therapy of Bowenoid papulosis and Bowen's disease. *J Dermatol Surg Oncol* 1986; **12**: 1253–7.

80 Robinson PJ, Carruth JA, Fairris GM. Photodynamic therapy: a better treatment for widespread Bowen's disease. *Br J Dermatol* 1988; **119**: 59–61.

81 Jones CM, Mang T, Cooper M, Wilson BD, Stoll HL Jr. Photodynamic therapy in the treatment of Bowen's disease. *J Am Acad Dermatol* 1992; **27**: 979–82.

82 Svanberg K, Andersson T, Killander D et al. Photodynamic therapy of non-melanoma malignant tumours of the skin using topical delta-amino levulinic acid sensitization and laser irradiation. *Br J Dermatol* 1994; **130**: 743–51.

83 Cairnduff F, Stringer MR, Hudson EJ, Ash

DV, Brown SB. Superficial photodynamic therapy with topical 5-aminolaevulinic acid for superficial primary and secondary skin cancer. *Br J Cancer* 1994; **69**: 605–8.

84 Stables GI, Stringer MR, Robinson DJ, Ash DV. The treatment of Bowen's disease by topical aminolaevulinic acid photodynamic therapy. *Br J Dermatol* 1998; **139 (Suppl. 51)**: 74.

85 Stables GI, Stringer MR, Robinson DJ, Ash DV. Large patches of Bowen's disease treated by topical aminolaevulinic acid photodynamic therapy. *Br J Dermatol* 1997; **136**: 957–60.

86 Stables GI, Stringer MR, Robinson DV, Ash DV. Topical amino-laevulinic acid photodynamic therapy for the treatment of erythroplasia of Queyrat. *Br J Dermatol* 1999; **140**: 514–517.

87 Varma S, Anstey A, Wilson H et al. Photodynamic therapy for the treatment of Bowen's disease, solar keratoses, and superficial basal cell carcinomas: 12 months experience with a novel light source. *Br J Dermatol* 1998; **139 (Suppl. 51)**: 19.

88 Blank AA, Schnyder UW. Soft-X-ray therapy in Bowen's disease and erythroplasia of Queyrat. *Dermatologica* 1985; **171**: 89–94.

89 Gordon KB, Roenick HH, Gendleman M. Treatment of multiple lesions of Bowen disease with isotretinoin and interferon alpha. *Arch Dermatol* 1997; **133**: 691–3.

90 Sonnex TS, Ralfs IG, de Plaza Lanza M, Dawber RP. Treatment of erythroplasia of Queyrat with liquid nitrogen cryosurgery. *Br J Dermatol* 1982; **106**: 581–4.

91 Papillon J, Chassard JL. Respective roles of radiotherapy and surgery in the management of epidermoid carcinoma of the anal margin. *Dis Colon Rectum* 1992; **35**: 422–9.

92 Baker EJ, Hobbs ER. Enhancement of the clinical margins of Bowen's disease by acetowhitening. *J Dermatol Surg Oncol* 1990; **16**: 846–50.

93 Schell BJ, Rosen T. Evaluation of acetowhitening in Bowen's disease. *J Dermatol Surg Oncol* 1990; **20**: 740–2.

Appendix 1. Strength of recommendations

A   There is good evidence to support the use of the procedure

B   There is fair evidence to support the use of the procedure

C   There is poor evidence to support the use of the procedure

D   There is fair evidence to support the rejection of the use of the procedure

E   There is good evidence to support the rejection of the use of the procedure

Appendix 2. Quality of evidence

I   Evidence obtained from at least one properly designed, randomized control trial

II–i Evidence obtained from well designed control trials without randomization

II–ii Evidence obtained from well designed cohort or case control analytic studies, preferably from more than one centre or research group

II–iii Evidence obtained from multiple time series with or without the intervention. Dramatic results in uncontrolled experiments (such as the results of the introduction of penicillin treatment in the 1940s) could also be regarded as this type of evidence

III   Opinions of respected authorities based on clinical experience, descriptive studies or reports of expert committees

IV   Evidence inadequate owing to problems of methodology (e.g. sample size, or length of comprehensiveness of follow-up or conflicts in evidence)

Appendix II
Guidelines for the management of basal cell carcinoma

NR Telfer, GB Colver and PW Bowers

Disclaimer

These guidelines on the management of basal cell carcinoma have been prepared for dermatologists on behalf of the British Association of Dermatologists. They present evidence-based guidance for treatment, with identification of the strength of evidence available at the time of preparation of the guidelines, and a brief overview of epidemiological aspects, diagnosis and investigation.

Definition

BCC is a slow-growing, locally invasive malignant epidermal skin tumour which mainly affects Caucasians. BCC tends to infiltrate tissues in a three-dimensional contiguous fashion through the irregular growth of subclinical finger-like outgrowths.[2] Metastasis is extremely rare,[3] and the morbidity associated with BCC is related to local tissue invasion and destruction, particularly on the head and neck. The clinical appearances and morphology are diverse, including nodular, cystic, ulcerated ('rodent ulcer'), superficial, morphoeic (sclerosing), keratotic and pigmented variants.

Incidence

BCC is the most common cancer in the U.S.A. and Australia[4] and is showing an increase in incidence in the U.K. The most significant aetiological factor is chronic exposure to ultraviolet light and consequently exposed areas such as the head and neck are the most commonly involved sites,[5] although increasing age, male sex and a tendency to freckle are also known risk factors.[4] BCCs may also arise in basal cell naevus (Gorlin's) syndrome and in organoid naevi. Once a person has developed a BCC there is a significantly increased risk of developing subsequent BCCs at other sites.[6-9]

Diagnostic tests

The treatment of many BCCs is based upon a clinical diagnosis. However, where clinical doubt exists, or when patients are referred for specialized forms of treatment a pre-operative biopsy is recommended. Biopsy will also provide information on the histological subtype of the BCC which has a direct bearing on the prognosis (Table 1).

Concept of 'low-risk' and 'high-risk' basal cell carcinomas

Individual tumours can be divided into relatively low- and high-risk categories by considering the recognized prognostic factors (Table 1). This will allow the clinician to select the most appropriate form(s) of treatment.

Additional factors

Once the tumour has been assessed the most appropriate treatment options can be discussed with the patient. Patients reluctant to consider any form of surgery are best referred for radiotherapy. Similarly, co-existing medical conditions or drug medication may influence the choice between surgical and non-surgical treatment. Not all BCCs require treatment; aggressive treatment might be inappropriate for patients of advanced age or poor general health, especially for asymptomatic low-risk lesions that are unlikely to cause significant morbidity. Furthermore, some elderly or frail patients with symptomatic or high-risk tumours might prefer less aggressive treatments designed to palliate rather than cure their tumours. Local availability of various specialized services, together with the experience and preferences of the

Table 1
Factors affecting the prognosis of basal cell carcinoma

Tumour size[2,11,12,27,28,34,40,41,48]
Tumour site[5,10–12,16,34,35,58,60]
Tumour type and definition of tumour margins[2,27,41]
Growth pattern/Histological subtype[2,41,42,75–79]
Failure of previous treatment (recurrent tumours)[2,15,17,37,41,50,77,80,81]
Immunocompromised patients[82]

dermatologist managing the case are also factors which will influence the selection of therapy.

Surgical techniques

The most commonly used surgical techniques can be divided into two main categories:

Destructive

Curettage and cautery/electrodesiccation. There are wide variations in how this technique is performed (e.g. type of curette used, number of cycles of treatment) and both experience in the technique[10] and appropriate selection of cases is crucial to success. Curettage and cautery is best used for selected low-risk lesions (small, well defined primary lesions with non-aggressive histology usually in non-critical sites[11–14] where 5-year cure rates of up to 97% are possible.[11] Curettage and cautery is generally not recommended for the management of recurrent[15] or morphoeic tumours, and tumours in 'high-risk' facial sites such as the nose, nasolabial folds and around the eyes,[10,12,13,16–18] although some reports suggest acceptable results for such tumours.[19]

Tumour size is an important factor as the recurrence rate rises dramatically with increasing tumour size.[20] (Strength of Evidence [Appendix] A, II–iii)

A literature review of all studies published since 1947 suggested an overall 5-year cure rate of 92´3% following curettage and cautery for primary BCC.[21] However, a similar review of all studies published since 1945 suggested an overall 5-year cure rate of 60% following curettage and cautery for recurrent BCC. This supports the view that curettage and cautery is much less useful in the treatment of recurrent BCC, especially in high-risk sites.[17] (Strength of Evidence A, II–ii)

Cryosurgery. Cryosurgery is widely used to treat solitary and multiple BCCs. Individual technique can vary considerably, using the open or closed spray techniques and single, double or triple freeze/thaw cycles.[22] Subcutaneous temperature monitoring using thermocouples is sometimes used.[23]

Many large published series specifically exclude the treatment of very high-risk BCCs, emphasizing the importance of careful selection of appropriate lesions with non-aggressive histology, away from critical facial sites in order to achieve high cure rates.[18,23,24–26] (Strength of Evidence A, II–ii)

There are reports in the ophthalmological literature[27–29] recommending the use of cryosurgery for periocular BCC, although full-thickness eyelid defects may occasionally result and require subsequent plastic surgical reconstruction.[27]

Thorough curettage immediately prior to cryosurgery may help to increase the cure rate.[30] (Strength of Evidence A, II–ii)

As with most treatment modalities, cryosurgery is less useful in the treatment of recurrent BCC.[21]

Post-operative wound care can be a problem. However, the treatment is usually well tolerated when performed on a local anaesthetic, outpatient basis[24] and the cosmetic results can be excellent.[31]

Carbon dioxide laser. Carbon dioxide (CO_2) laser surgery is not a widely used form of treatment and there is little published follow-up data to date. The treatment is mainly recommended for low-risk lesions. When combined with curettage, CO_2 laser surgery may be useful in the treatment of large or multiple superficial BCCs.[32,33]

Excisional

Excision with predetermined margins. The primary objective of any excisional procedure is to remove the tumour entirely. However, there is a confusing literature suggesting that total removal of some BCCs may not be necessary to effect cure. This will be discussed further under the section on management of incompletely excised BCC (positive histological margins).

Discussion of the surgical excision of BCC is divided into the following sections:

1   Primary (previously untreated) BCC. Surgical excision is a highly effective treatment for primary BCC.[34–36] (Strength of Evidence A, II-ii) The excised tissue can be examined histologically[37,38] and the peripheral and deep surgical margins can be grossly assessed. The overall cosmetic results are usually good. The use of thorough curettage prior to excision of primary BCC may help to increase the cure rate by more accurately defining the true borders of the BCC.[39] The size of the surgical margins should correlate with the likelihood that subclinical tumour extensions exist (Table 1). Few data exist on the

correct deep surgical margin as this will depend upon the local anatomy. In an average case, excision will extend deeply through subcutaneous fat. Studies using horizontal frozen sectioning•Mohs' micrographic surgery (MMS)•to detect accurately BCC at any part of the surgical margin suggest that, for a small (< 20 mm) well defined BCC 3 mm peripheral surgical margins will clear the tumour in 85% of cases, and a 4–5 mm margin will increase the peripheral clearance rate to approximately 95%, i.e. approximately 5% of small, well-defined BCCs show subclinical spread of > 4mm.[2,40] In contrast to small primary BCCs, morphoeic and large BCCs require wider surgical margins for complete histological resection. For primary morphoeic BCC, the rate of complete excision with increasing peripheral surgical margins is as follows: 3 mm margin: 66%, 5 mm margin: 82%, 13–15 mm margin: > 95%.[2]

2   Recurrent (previously treated) BCC. The results of all published series on the surgical excision of BCC show that cure rates for recurrent BCC are inferior to those for primary lesions.[17] Recurrent BCCs require wider peripheral surgical margins than primary lesions with or without standard (non-Mohs) frozen section control.[37] Peripheral excision margins for recurrent BCC of 5–10 mm have been suggested.[41] (Strength of Evidence A, II-ii)

3   Incompletely excised BCC (positive histological margins). The management of incompletely excised BCC remains controversial. Some evidence suggests that the total removal of some BCCs may not be necessary to effect cure and that up to two thirds of incompletely excised BCCs that are not re-treated do not recur.[42,43] This raises a series of questions.

(a) Do incompletely excised (positive margin) BCCs contain residual tumour? A study in which 43 incompletely excised BCCs were re-excised and the tissue examined using standard tissue sectioning techniques suggested that only 7% contained residual BCC.[44] However, when 78 incompletely excised BCCs were re-excised and examined using horizontal frozen sectioning (MMS) in order to detect BCC more accurately at any part of the surgical margin, 55% were found to contain residual BCC.[45] (Strength of Evidence A, II-iii)

(b) Do incompletely excised (positive margin) BCCs recur if they are not retreated? In a prospective study of 34 incompletely excised BCCs, 41% recurred after a mean follow-up of 2 years.[46] In a review of 60 incompletely excised BCCs, 35 (58%) recurred.[47] In a series of 187 incompletely excised BCCs, with 93% occurring on the head and neck, 119 were immediately retreated with radiotherapy, one was excised and 67 were not treated. After a median follow-up period of 2´7 years, statistical analysis suggested a 5-year probability of cure in the radiotherapy group of 91%, and in the untreated group of 61%.[48]

(c) Does it matter which surgical margin(s) are involved with tumour? In a review of 60 incompletely excised BCCs, 35 (58%) recurred.[47] The risk of recurrence was highest in those lesions where both lateral and deep margins were involved with BCC and when the incomplete excision was performed to remove recurrent BCC, especially following radiation therapy.[47] BCCs incompletely excised at the deep margin were considered especially difficult to cure with re-excision.[47] Other authors have calculated that the probability of recurrence of incompletely excised BCC varies when only the lateral margins were involved (17% risk of recurrence) and if the deep margins were involved (33% risk of recurrence).[48]

(d) Should incompletely excised (positive margin) BCCs be retreated? Several studies have strongly recommended the immediate re-treatment of incompletely excised BCC[45–47,49] especially those where the surgical defect has been repaired using skin flaps or skin grafts.[50] Overall, an expectant policy would be most appropriate for BCCs that are incompletely excised on a lateral margin only, are of non-aggressive histological type, were not previously recurrent tumours, and involve non-critical anatomical sites. In contrast, it seems most appropriate to re-treat BCCs that are incompletely excised on the deep margin, are of an aggressive histological type, were previously recurrent tumours and involve critical anatomical sites. In this latter situation, re-excision with or without frozen section control or MMS are probably the treatments of choice (Table 2).

Mohs' micrographic surgery

MMS[51–57] offers highly accurate yet conservative removal of BCC. It offers high cure rates for even the most difficult of BCCs[58] together with the maximal preservation of normal tissues. The indications for using MMS are summarized in Table 2. (Strength of Evidence A, II-i)

A review of all studies published since 1947 suggested an overall 5-year cure rate of 99% following MMS for primary BCC[21] and a review of all studies published since 1945 suggested an overall 5-year cure rate of 94´4% following MMS for recurrent BCC.[17] MMS is a relatively specialized treatment, is relatively expensive when compared with other outpatient-based treatments for BCC, and is undoubtedly time-consuming.

Non-surgical techniques

Radiotherapy

Radiotherapy (RT) is an extremely useful form of treatment,[48,59,60] but faces the same problem of accurately identifying tumour margins as standard excisional surgery. RT includes a range of treatments using different types of equipment, each with its own specific indications and side-effects. It is, therefore best performed by clinical oncologists with a specialist interest in skin cancer. Collaboration between dermatologists, plastic surgeons and clinical oncologists in the management of patients with high-risk BCC is a common and valuable feature of dermatological care in the U.K. (Strength of Evidence A, II-i)

Careful patient selection can result in very high cure rates; in a series of 412 BCCs treated with RT, 5-year cure rates of 90´3% were achieved.[34] In a prospective trial, where 93

Table 2
Basal cell carcinoma (BCC), indications for Mohs' micrographic surgery

Site
    Eyes, ears, lips, nose, nasolabial folds[54,55,79,83]
Histological subtype
    Morphoeic, infiltrative, micronodular
Recurrent BCCs[17,83]
Size
    > 2 cm, especially in high-risk sites[17,21,41,55,63,77,83–90]
Special situations
    Perineural spread[91]

patients with BCC were randomized to receive either cryosurgery or radiation therapy; the 2-year cure rate for the RT group was 96%.[26] A review of all studies published since 1947 suggested an overall 5-year cure rate of 91·3% following RT for primary BCC,[21] and a review of all studies published since 1945 suggested an overall 5-year cure rate of 90·2% following RT for recurrent BCC.[17]

Radiotherapy can be used to treat many types of BCC, even those overlying bone and cartilage, although it is probably less suitable for the treatment of large tumours in critical sites, as very large BCC masses are often both resistant and require radiation doses that closely approach tissue tolerance.[61] It is also not indicated for BCCs on areas subject to repeated trauma such as the extremities or trunk[61] and for young patients as the late-onset changes of cutaneous atrophy and telangiectasis may result in a cosmetic result inferior to that following surgery.[59] It can also be difficult to use RT to re-treat BCCs that have recurred following RT. Modern fractionated dose therapy has many advantages but requires multiple visits to a specialist centre.[62] Lateonset fibrosis may cause problems such as epiphora and ectropion following treatment of lower eyelid and inner canthal lesions, where cataract formation is also a recognized risk,[62] although this can be minimized by the use of protective contact lenses.

There is some suggestion that BCCs recurring following RT may behave in a particularly aggressive and infiltrative fashion,[47,63,64] although this may simply reflect that these lesions were of an aggressive, high-risk type from the very beginning.

Topical therapy

This mainly involves topical 5-fluorouracil (5FU). Treatment is especially useful for low-risk, extrafacial BCC but it cannot be expected to eradicate invasive BCC or lesions with follicular involvement.[65] Topical 5FU therapy can be particularly helpful in the management of multiple superficial BCCs on the trunk and lower limbs. (Strength of Evidence A, II–ii)

Intralesional interferon

In a pilot study of low-risk BCCs, thrice-weekly intralesional injections of human recombinant interferon a2 (IFN-a2) were given for 3 weeks with histological evidence of tumour clearance.[66] The same authors later reported a placebo-controlled study in which 172 nodular or superficial BCCs were treated with intralesional IFN-a2, resulting in a 14% immediate treatment failure rate and a 19% recurrence rate at 1 year.[67] Other studies have confirmed a 20%[68] to 45%[69] failure rate 3 months following treatment. Treatment of BCC with intralesional IFN-a2 is still essentially investigational and is unlikely to prove useful in high-risk tumours. It is also very expensive, time consuming and long-term cure rates are not yet available. (Strength of Evidence C, II–iii)

Photodynamic therapy

The use of topical photodynamic therapy (PDT) in the management of BCC is still essentially investigational and is not widely available in the U.K. In a study of 151 BCCs treated with PDT without long-term follow-up, 88% demonstrated a complete response.[70] (Strength of Evidence C, II-iii) Long-term follow-up data on large series is needed to demonstrate whether or not topical PDT has a role in the management of BCC. However, as depth of penetration of the photosensitizer appears to be a limiting factor with topical PDT,[71] it is only likely to be of benefit for the treatment of superficial BCC in low risk areas.[72] (Strength of Evidence C, III)

Chemotherapy

Chemotherapy has been used both for the management of uncontrolled local disease and for patients with metastatic BCC,[73] which is both an extremely rare and a rapidly fatal condition.[3]

Palliative therapy

In the debilitated patient aggressive treatment may be inappropriate for asymptomatic or low-risk BCC. Otherwise, palliative (non-curative) treatment may be appropriate, using simple debulking procedures or RT to gain local control of the BCC and improve the quality of life in the short term.

Retinoids

Oral retinoid therapy may prevent or delay the development of new BCCs. Such therapy has mainly been used in patients with the basal cell naevus (Gorlin's) syndrome and may also have a lesser effect in producing partial regression of existing BCCs.[74] Unfortunately, the relatively high doses necessary mean that compliance may be poor, and relapse occurs following the discontinuation of treatment.[74] (Strength of Evidence B, III)

Follow-up

Long-term hospital-based follow-up of all patients after treatment of BCC is neither necessary nor recommended. However, follow-up can be important for selected patients, although there is no clear consensus on either the frequency or total duration or such review. The main arguments for follow up are: (i) early detection of tumour recurrence; (ii) early detection and treatment of new lesions; and (iii) patient education, especially regarding sun protection measures. Most evidence suggests that the majority of BCCs which recur will present within 5 years of treatment,[75] although up to 18% will recur after this.[21] A review of all studies published since 1947 suggested that for primary (previously untreated) BCCs treated by a variety of modalities less than one-third of all recurrences occurred in the first year following treatment, 50% appear within 2 years, and 66% within 3 years.[21] Patients who have had one BCC are at significantly higher risk of developing new primary lesions,[6–8] many of which may go unnoticed by patients. In a 5-year prospective follow-up study of 1000 patients following treatment for BCC, 36% developed new primary BCCs[9] and 20% of patients with very fair skin types and frequent sun exposure went on to develop multiple BCCs.[9] Consequently, some authors have recommended long-term, even lifetime follow-up, particularly for patients with high-risk or multiple lesions.[8,21]

The early detection and appropriate re-treatment of either recurrent BCCs or new primary BCCs may help to increase the chances of permanent cure and to minimize morbidity. Patient education together with close collaboration with colleagues in primary care should allow the vast majority of adequately treated patients to be discharged back to the care of their general practitioners.

The relative value of the available forms of therapy for BCCs of different sizes, clinical and histological subtypes and involving both

Table 3

Primary (previously untreated) basal cell carcinoma: influence of tumour type, size (large ≥ 2 cm) and site on the selection of available forms of treatment

Basal cell carcinoma • histology • size • site	Topical therapy including photo-dynamic therapy	Curettage and cautery	Radiation therapy	Cryo-surgery	Excision	Mohs micro-graphic surgery
Superficial, small and low-risk site	*	**	?	**	?	×
Nodular, small and low-risk site	–	**	?	**	***	×
Morphoeic, small and low-risk site	–	*	*	*	***	?
Superficial, large and low-risk site	*	**	*	***	*	?
Nodular, large and low-risk site	×	**	**	**	***	?
Morphoeic, large and low-risk site	×	–	*	*	***	**
Superficial, small and high-risk site	×	*	**	**	***	*
Nodular, small and high-risk site	×	*	**	**	***	**
Morphoeic, small and high-risk site	×	–	*	*	**	***
Superficial, large and high-risk site	×	–	**	*	**	**
Nodular, large and high-risk site	×	×	**	*	**	***
Morphoeic, large and high risk site	×	×	*	×	*	***

***, Probable treatment of choice; **, generally good choice; *, generally fair choice; ?, reasonable, but not often needed; –, generally poor choice; ×, probably should not be used.

Table 4

Recurrent BCC: influence of tumour type, size (large ≥ 2 cm) and site on the selection of available forms of treatment

Basal cell carcinoma • histology • size • site	Topical therapy including photo-dynamic therapy	Curettage and cautery	Radiation therapy	Cryo-surgery	Excision	Mohs micro-graphic surgery
Superficial, small and low-risk site	×	*	*	**	***	?
Nodular, small and low-risk site	×	**	**	**	***	?
Morphoeic, small and low-risk site	×	–	**	**	***	*
Superficial, large and low-risk site	×	*	**	***	*	*
Nodular, large and low-risk site	×	–	*	*	***	*
Morphoeic, large and low-risk site	×	–	*	*	**	**
Superficial, small and high-risk site	×	–	*	*	**	**
Nodular, small and high-risk site	×	–	*	*	***	**
Morphoeic, small and high-risk site	×	×	*	*	**	***
Superficial, large and high-risk site	×	×	*	–	**	**
Nodular, large and high-risk site	×	×	*	–	**	***
Morphoeic, large and high-risk site	×	×	*	–	*	***

***, Probable treatment of choice; **, generally good choice; *, generally fair choice; ?, reasonable, but not often needed; –, generally poor choice; ×, probably should not be used.

high- and low-risk body sites are summarized in Table 3 (primary BCCs) and Table 4 (recurrent BCCs).

Appendix

Table A1
Strength of recommendations

A There is good evidence to support the use of the procedure
B There is fair evidence to support the use of the procedure
C There is poor evidence to support the use of the procedure
D There is fair evidence to support the rejection of the use of the procedure
E There is good evidence to support the rejection of the use of the procedure

Table A2
Quality of evidence

I	Evidence obtained from at least one properly designed, randomized control trial
II–i	Evidence obtained from well-designed controlled trials without randomization
II–ii	Evidence obtained from well-designed cohort or case–control analytic studies, preferably from more than one centre or research group
II–iii	Evidence obtained from multiple time series with or without the intervention. Dramatic results in uncontrolled experiments (such as the introduction of penicillin treatment in the 1940s) could be regarded as this type of evidence
III	Opinions of respected authorities based on clinical experience, descriptive studies or reports of expert committees
IV	Evidence inadequate owing to problems of methodology (e.g. sample size, or length or comprehensiveness of follow-up or conflicts of evidence)

References

1 Albright SD. Treatment of skin cancer using multiple modalities. *J Am Acad Dermatol* 1982; **197**: 143–71.

2 Breuninger H, Dietz K. Prediction of subclinical tumor infiltration in basal cell carcinoma. *J Dermatol Surg Oncol* 1991; **17**: 574–8.

3 Lo JS, Snow SN, Reizner GT et al. Metastatic basal cell carcinoma report of twelve cases with a review of the literature. *J Am Acad Dermatol* 1991; **24**: 715–19.

4 Gilbody JS, Aitken J, Green A. What causes basal cell carcinoma to be the commonest cancer? *Aust J Public Health* 1994; **18**: 218–21.

5 Roenigk RK, Ratz JL, Bailin PL, Wheeland RG. Trends in the presentation and treatment of basal cell carcinomas. *J Dermatol Surg Oncol* 1986; **12**: 860–5.

6 Karagas MR, Stukel TA, Greenberg ER et al. Risk of subsequent basal cell carcinoma and squamous cell carcinoma of the skin among patients with prior skin cancer. Skin cancer prevention study group. *JAMA* 1992; **267**: 3305–10.

7 Schreiber MM, Moon TE, Fox SH, Davidson J. The risk of developing subsequent nonmelanoma skin cancers. *J Am Acad Dermatol* 1990; **23**: 1114–18.

8 Marghoob A, Kopf AW, Bart RS et al. Risk of another basal cell carcinoma developing after treatment of a basal cell carcinoma. *J Am Acad Dermatol* 1993; **28**: 22–8.

9 Robinson JK. Risk of developing another basal cell carcinoma. *Cancer* 1987; **60**: 118–20.

10 Kopf AW, Bart RS, Schrager D, Lazar M, Popkin GL. Curettage–electrodesiccation treatment of basal cell carcinomas. *Arch Dermatol* 1977; **113**: 439–43.

11 Spiller WF, Spiller RF. Treatment of basal cell epithelioma by curettage and electrodesiccation. *J Am Acad Dermatol* 1984; **11**: 808–14.

12 Silverman MK, Kopf AW, Grin CM, Bart RS, Levenstein MJ. Recurrence rates of treated basal cell carcinomas. Part 2: Curettage–electrodesiccation. *J Dermatol Surg Oncol* 1991; **17**: 720–6.

13 Sughe-d'Aubermont PC, Bennett RG. Failure of curettage and electrodesiccation for removal of basal cell carcinoma. *Arch Dermatol* 1984; **120**: 1456–60.

14 Salasche SJ. Status of curettage and desiccation in the treatment of primary basal cell carcinoma. *J Am Acad Dermatol* 1984; **10**: 285– 7.

15 Menn H, Robins P, Kopf AW, Bart RS. The recurrent basal cell epithelioma. A study of 100 cases of recurrent, re-treated basal cell epitheliomas. *Arch Dermatol* 1974; **103**: 628–31.

16 Salasche SJ. Curettage and electrodesiccation in the treatment of midfacial basal cell epithelioma. *J Am Acad Dermatol* 1983; **8**: 496–503.

17 Rowe DE, Carroll RJ, Day CL Jr. Mohs surgery is the treatment of choice for recurrent (previously treated) basal cell carcinoma. *J Dermatol Surg Oncol* 1989; **15**: 424–31.

18 Nordin P, Larko O, Stenquist B. Five-year results of curettage–cryosurgery of selected large primary basal cell carcinomas on the nose: an alternative treatment in a geographical area underserved by Mohs' surgery. *Br J Dermatol* 1997; **136**: 180–3.

19 Whelan CS, Deckers PJ. Electrocoagulation for skin cancer: an old oncological tool revisited. *Cancer* 1981; **47**: 2280–7.

20 Sweet RD. The management of basal cell carcinoma by curettage. *Br J Dermatol* 1983; **75**: 137–48.

21 Rowe DE, Carroll RJ, Day CL Jr. Long-term recurrence rates in previously untreated (primary) basal cell carcinoma: implications for patient follow-up. *J Dermatol Surg Oncol* 1989; **15**: 315–28.

22 Graham G. Statistical data on malignant tumors in cryosurgery: 1982. *J Dermatol Surg Oncol* 1983; **9**: 238–9.

23 Zacarian SA. Cryosurgery of cutaneous carcinomas. An 18 year study of 3022 patients with 4228 carcinomas. *J Am Acad Dermatol* 1983; **9**: 947–56.

24 Holt PJ. Cryotherapy for skin cancer: results over a 5 year period using liquid nitrogen spray cryosurgery. *Br J Dermatol* 1988; **119**: 231–40.

25 Kuflik EG, Gage AA. The five-year cure rate achieved by cryosurgery for skin cancer. *J Am Acad Dermatol* 1991; **24**: 1002–4.

26 Hall VL, Leppard BJ, McGill J et al. Treatment of basal cell carcinoma: comparison of radiotherapy and cryotherapy. *Clin Radiol* 1986; **37**: 33–4.

27 Fraunfelder FT, Zacarian SA, Limmer BL, Wingfield D. Cryosurgery for malignancies of the eyelid. *Ophthalmology* 1980; **87**: 461–5.

28 Fraunfelder FT, Zacarian SA, Wingfield DL, Limmer BL. Results of cryotherapy for eyelid malignancies. *Am J Ophthalmol* 1984; **97**: 184–8.

29 Gunnarson G, Larko O, Hersle K. Cryosurgery of eyelid basal cell carcinomas. *Acta Opthalmol Copenh* 1990; **68**: 241–5.

30 Spiller WF, Spiller RF. Treatment of basal cell carcinomas by a combination of curettage and cryosurgery. *J Dermatol Surg Oncol* 1997; **3**: 443–7.

31 McIntosh GS, Osborne DR, Li AK, Hobbs KE. Basal cell carcinoma: a review of treatment results with special reference to cryotherapy. *Postgrad Med J* 1983; **59**: 698–701.

32 Wheland RG, Bailin PL, Roenigk RK, Ratz JL. Carbon dioxide laser vaporization and curettage in the treatment of large or multiple superficial basal cell carcinomas. *J Dermatol Surg Oncol* 1987; **13**: 119–25.

33 Bandieramonte G, Lepera P, Moglia D, Bono A, De-Vecchi C, Milani F. Laser microsurgery for superficial T1-T2 basal cell carcinoma of the eyelid margins. *Ophthalmology* 1997; **104**: 1179–84.

34 Dubin N, Kopf AW. Multivariate risk score for recurrence of cutaneous basal cell

carcinomas. *Arch Dermatol* 1983; **119**: 373–7.

35 Bart RS, Schrager D, Kopf AW, Bromberg J, Dubin N. Scalpel excision of basal cell carcinomas. *Arch Dermatol* 1978; **114**: 739– 42.

36 Marchac D, Papadopoulos O, Duport G. Curative and aesthetic results of surgical treatment of 138 basal cell carcinomas. *J Dermatol Surg Oncol* 1982; **8**: 379–87.

37 Cataldo PA, Stoddard PB, Reed WP. Use of frozen section analysis in the treatment of basal cell carcinoma. *Am J Surg* 1990; **159**: 561–3.

38 Chalfin J, Putterman AM. Frozen section control in the surgery of basal cell carcinoma of the eyelid. *Am J Ophthalmol* 1979; **87**: 802–9.

39 Johnson TM, Tromovitch TA, Swanson NA. Combined curettage and excision: a treatment method for primary basal cell carcinoma. *J Am Acad Dermatol* 1991; **24**: 613–17.

40 Wolf DJ, Zitelli JA. Surgical margins for basal cell carcinoma. *Arch Dermatol* 1987; **123**: 340–4.

41 Burg G, Hirsch RD, Konz B, Braun-Falco O. Histographic surgery: accuracy of visual assessment of the margins of basal-cell epithelioma. *J Dermatol Surg Oncol* 1975; **1**: 21–4.

42 Dellon AL, DeSilva S, Connolly M, Ross A. Prediction of recurrence in incompletely excised basal cell carcinoma. *Plast Reconstr Surg* 1985; **75**: 860–71.

43 Gooding CA, White G, Yatsuhashi M. Significance of marginal extension in excised basal cell carcinoma. *N Engl J Med* 1965; **273**: 923–4.

44 Sarma DP, Griffing CC, Weilbaecher TG. Observations on the inadequately excised basal cell carcinoma. *J Surg Oncol* 1984; **25**: 79–80.

45 Bieley HC, Kirsner RS, Reyes BA, Garland LD. The use of Mohs micrographic surgery for determination of residual tumour in incompletely excised basal cell carcinoma. *J Am Acad Dermatol* 1992; **26**: 754–6.

46 DeSilva SP, Dellon AL. Recurrence rate of positive margin basal cell carcinoma results of a five-year prospective study. *J Surg Oncol* 1985; **28**: 72–4.

47 Richmond JD, Davie RM. The significance of incomplete excision in patients with basal cell carcinoma. *Br J Plast Surg* 1987; **40**: 63–7. 48 Liu FF, Maki R, Warde P, Payne D, Fitzpatrick P. A management approach to incompletely excised basal cell carcinomas of skin. *Int J Radiat Oncol Biol Phys* 1991; **20**: 423–8.

49 Hauben DJ, Zirkin H, Mahler D, Sacks M. The biologic behavior of basal cell carcinoma: Part I. *Plast Reconstr Surg* 1982; **69**: 103–9.

50 Koplin L, Zarem HA. Recurrent basal cell carcinoma: a review concerning the incidence, behavior, and management of recurrent basal cell carcinoma, with emphasis on the incompletely excised lesion. *Plast Reconstr Surg* 1980; **65**: 656–64.

51 Mohs FE. Chemosurgery: a microscopically controlled method of cancer excision. *Arch Surg* 1941; **42**: 279–95.

52 Mohs FE. Chemosurgery for skin cancer: fixed tissue and fresh tissue techniques. *Arch Dermatol* 1976; **112**: 211–15.

53 Robins P. Chemosurgery; my 15 years of experience. *J Dermatol Surg Oncol* 1981; **7**: 779–89.

54 Tromovitch TA, Beirne G, Beirne C. Mohs technique (cancer chemosurgery) treatment of recurrent cutaneous carcinomas. *Cancer* 1966; **19**: 867–8.

55 Tromovitch TA, Stegman SJ. Microscope-controlled excision of cutaneous tumors: chemosurgery, fresh tissue technique. *Cancer* 1978; **41**: 653–8.

56 Cottel WI, Bailin PL, Albom MJ et al. Essentials of Mohs micrographic surgery. *J Dermatol Surg Oncol* 1988; **14**: 11–13.

57 Dzubow LM. Mohs surgery. *Lancet* 1994; **343**: 433–4.

58 Robins P, Reyes BA. Cure rates of skin cancer treated by Mohs micrographic surgery. In Dermatologic Surgery: Principles and Practice

(Roenigk RK, Roenigk HH Jr, eds). New York: Marcel Dekker, 1989; 853–8.

59   Silverman MK, Kopf AW, Gladstein AH, Bart RS, Grin CM, Levenstein MJ. Recurrence rates of treated basal cell carcinomas. Part 4: X-ray therapy. *J Dermatol Surg Oncol* 1992; **18**: 549–54.

60   Silverman MK, Kopf AW, Bart RS, Grin CM, Levenstein MJ. Recurrence rates of treated basal cell carcinomas. Part 3: Surgical excision. *J Dermatol Surg Oncol* 1992; **18**: 471–6.

61   Cooper JS. Radiotherapy in the treatment of skin cancers. In: Cancer of the Skin (Friedman RJ, Rigel DS, Kopf AW, Harris MN, Baker D, eds.) Philadelphia: WB Saunders 1991; 553–68.

62   Orton CI. The treatment of basal cell carcinoma by radiotherapy. *Clin Oncol* 1978; **4**: 317–22.

63   Smith SP, Grande DJ. Basal cell carcinoma recurring after radiotherapy: a unique difficult treatment subclass of recurrent basal cell carcinoma. *J Dermatol Surg Oncol* 1991; **17**: 26–30.

64   Smith SP, Foley EH, Grande DJ. Use of Mohs micrographic surgery to establish quantitative proof of heightened tumor spread in basal cell carcinoma recurrent following radiotherapy. *J Dermatol Surg Oncol* 1990; **16**: 1012–16.

65   Goette DK. Tropical chemotherapy with 5-fluorouracil. A review. *J Am Acad Dermatol* 1981; **4**: 633–6.

66   Greenway HT, Cornell RC, Tanner DJ et al. Treatment of basal cell carcinoma with intralesional interferon. *J Am Acad Dermatol* 1986; **15**: 437–40.

67   Cornell RC, Greenway HT, Tucker SB et al. Intralesional interferon therapy for basal cell carcinoma. *J Am Acad Dermatol* 1990; **23**: 694–700.

68   Edwards L, Tucker SB, Perednia D et al. The effect of an intralesional sustained-release formulation of interferon alfa2b on basal cell carcinomas. *Arch Dermatol* 1990; **126**: 1029– 32.

69   Healsmith MF, Berth Jones J, Fletcher A, Graham Brown RA. Treatment of basal cell carcinoma with intralesional interferon alpha-2b. *J R Soc Med* 1991; **84**: 524–6.

70   Wilson BD, Mang TS, Stoll H et al. Photodynamic therapy for the treatment of basal cell carcinoma. *Arch Dermatol* 1992; **128**: 1597–601.

71   Morton CA, MacKie RM, Whitehurst C, Moore JV, McColl JH. Photodynamic therapy for basal cell carcinoma: effect of tumor thickness and duration of photosensitizer application on response. *Arch Dermatol* 1998; **134**: 248–9.

72   Peng Q, Warloe T, Berg K et al. 5-Aminolevulinic acid-based photodynamic therapy. Clinical research and future challenges. *Cancer* 1997; **79**: 2282–308.

73   Guthrie TH Jr, Porubsky ES, Luxenberg MN et al. Cisplatin-based chemotherapy in advanced basal and squamous cell carcinomas of the skin: results in 28 patients including 13 patients receiving multimodality therapy. *J Clin Oncol* 1990; **8**: 342–6.

74   Hodak E, Ginzburg A, David M et al. Etretinate treatment of nevoid basal cell carcinoma syndrome. Therapeutic and chemopreventive effect. *Int J Dermatol* 1987; **26**: 606–9.

75   Hauben DJ, Zirkin H, Mahler D, Sacks M. The biologic behavior of basal cell carcinoma: analysis of recurrence in excised basal cell carcinoma: Part II. *Plast Reconstr Surg* 1982; **69**: 110–16.

76   Sexton M, Jones DB, Maloney ME. Histologic pattern analysis of basal cell carcinoma. Study of a series of 1039 consecutive neoplasms. *J Am Acad Dermatol* 1990; **23**: 1118–26.

77   Lang PG Jr, Maize JC. Histologic evolution of recurrent basal cell carcinomas and treatment implications. *J Am Acad Dermatol* 1986; **14**: 186–96.

78   Salasche SJ, Amonette RA. Morpheaform basal-cell epitheliomas: a study of subclinical extensions in a series of 51 cases. *J Dermatol Surg Oncol* 1981; **7**: 387–94.

79 Sloane JP. The value of typing basal cell carcinomas in predicting recurrence after surgical excision. *Br J Dermatol* 1977; **96**: 127– 32.

80 Silverman MK, Kopf AW, Grin CM, Bart RS, Levenstein MJ. recurrence rates of treated basal cell carcinomas. Part 1: Overview. *J Dermatol Surg Oncol* 1991; **17**: 713–18.

81 Sakura CY, Calamel PM. Comparison of treatment modalities for recurrent basal cell carcinoma. *Plast Reconstr Surg* 1979; **63**: 492–6.

82 Weimar VM, Ceiley RI, Goeken JA. Aggressive biologic behavior of basal and squamous cell cancers in patients with chronic lymphocytic leukemia or chronic lymphocytic lymphoma. *J Dermatol Surg Oncol* 1979; **5**: 609–14.

83 Mohs FE. Carcinoma of the skin: a summary of therapeutic results. In: Chemosurgery: Microscopically Controlled Surgery for Skin Cancer. Springfield, IL: Charles C Thomas, 1978; 153–64.

84 Mohs FE. Micrographic surgery for the microscopically controlled excision of eyelid cancers. *Arch Ophthalmol* 1986; **104**: 9 01–9.

85 Leshin B, Yeatts P, Anscher M et al. Management of periocular basal cell carcinoma: Mohs'; micrographic surgery versis radiotherapy. *Surv Ophthalmol* 1993; **38**: 193–212.

86 Riefkohl T, Pollack S, Georgiade GS. A rationale for the treatment of difficult basal cell and squamous cell carcinomas of the skin. *Ann Plast Surg* 1985; **15**: 99–104.

87 Ceilley RI, Anderson RL. Microscopically controlled excision of malignant neoplasms around eyelids followed by immediate surgical reconstruction. *J Dermatol Surg Oncol* 1978; **4**: 55–62.

88 Swanson NA, Grekin RC, Baker SR. Mohs' surgery: techniques, indications, and applications in head and neck surgery. *Head Neck Surg* 1983; **6**: 683–92.

89 Baker SR, Swanson NA. Management of nasal cutaneous malignant neoplasms: an interdisciplinary approach. *Arch Otolaryngol* 1983; **109**: 473–9.

90 Peters CR, Dinner MI, Dolsky RL, Bailin PL, Hardy RW. The combined multidisciplinary approach to invasive basal cell tumours of the scalp. *Ann Plast Surg* 1980; **4**: 199–204.

91 Hanke CW, Wolf RL, Hochman SA et al. Perineural spread of basal cell carcinoma. *J Dermatol Surg Oncol* 1983; **9**: 742–5.

Appendix III
Multiprofessional guidelines for the management of the patient with primary cutaneous squamous cell carcinoma

R Motley, P Kersey, C Lawrence, on behalf of the British Association of Dermatologists, the British Association of Plastic Surgeons, and the Faculty of Clinical Oncology of the Royal College of Radiologists

Summary

These guidelines for management of primary cutaneous squamous cell carcinoma present evidence-based guidance for treatment, with identification of the strength of evidence available at the time of preparation of the guidelines, and a brief overview of epidemiological aspects, diagnosis and investigation.

Disclaimer

These guidelines, prepared on behalf of the British Association of Dermatologists, the British Association of Plastic Surgeons and in consultation with members of the Faculty of Clinical Oncology of the Royal College of Radiologists, reflect the best published data available at the time the report was prepared. Caution should be exercised in interpreting the data; the results of future studies may require alteration of the conclusions or recommenda-tions in this report. It may be necessary or even desirable to depart from the guidelines in the interests of specific patients and special circumstances. Just as adherence to the guide-lines may not constitute defence against a claim of negligence, so deviation from them should not be necessarily deemed negligent.

Footnote

These guidelines were commissioned by the British Association of Dermatologists Therapy Guidelines and Audit subcommittee. Members of the committee are NH Cox (Chairman), AV Anstey, CB Bunker, MJD Goodfield, AS Highet, D Mehta, RH Meyrick Thomas, JK Schofield. The Multiprofessional Skin Cancer Committee representing the British Associa-tion of Dermatologists, the British Association of Plastic Surgeons and members of the Faculty of Clinical Oncology of the Royal College of Radiologists consisted of: NH Cox,

AY Finlay, BR Allen, DS Murray, RW Griffiths, A Batchelor, D Morgan, JK Schofield, CB Bunker, NR Telfer, GB Colver, PW Bowers, DLL Roberts, A. Anstey, RJ Barlow, JA Newton-Bishop, ME Gore, N Kirkham and the authors.

Definition

Primary cutaneous squamous cell carcinoma (SCC) is a malignant tumour which may arise from the keratinizing cells of the epidermis or its appendages. It is locally invasive and has the potential to metastasize to other organs of the body. These guidelines are confined to the treatment of SCC of the skin and the vermilion border of the lip, and exclude SCC of the penis, vulva and anus, SCC *in situ* (Bowen's disease), SCC arising from mucous membranes and keratoacanthoma.

Incidence, aetiology and prevention

SCC is the second most common skin cancer and, in many countries, its incidence is rising.[1–5] Its occurrence is usually related to chronic ultraviolet light exposure and is therefore especially common in the sun-damaged skin of fair-skinned individuals, in albinos and in those with xeroderma pigmentosum. It may develop *de novo*, as a result of previous exposure to ionizing radiation or arsenic, within chronic wounds, scars, burns, ulcers or sinus tracts, and from pre-existing lesions such as Bowen's disease ('intraepidermal SCC').[6–14] Individuals with impaired immune function, for example those receiving immunosuppressive drugs following allogeneic organ trans-plantation or those with lymphoma or leukaemia, are at increased risk of this tumour; some SCCs are associated with human papillomavirus infection.[15–23] There is good evidence linking SCCs with chronic actinic damage and to support the use of sun avoidance, protective clothing and effective sunblocks in the prevention of actinic keratoses and SCCs, and this is particularly important for patients receiving long term immunosuppressive medication.[24–27]

Clinical presentation

SCC usually presents as an indurated nodular keratinizing or crusted tumour which may ulcerate, or it may present as an ulcer without evidence of keratinization.

Diagnosis

The diagnosis is established histologically. The histology report should include the following: pathological pattern (for example 'adenoid type') cell morphology (for example 'spindle cell SCC'), degree of differentiation ('well differentiated' or 'poorly differentiated)', histological grade (as described by Broders, Appendix 2), depth (thickness in cm), the level of dermal invasion (as Clark's levels – excluding layers of surface keratin), and the presence or absence of perineural, vascular or lymphatic invasion. The margins of the excised tissue should be stained prior to tissue preparation to allow their identification histologically and comment should be made on the lateral and deep margins of excision.[28–40]

Prognosis

The accumulated experience of treating cutaneous SCC by various methods has allowed some generalizations to be made about prognosis based on the original lesion. Factors which influence metastatic potential include anatomical site, size, rate of growth, aetiology, degree of histological differentiation and host immunosuppression. These details are frequently omitted from reported series of treated SCC and the conclusions of such series must therefore be interpreted with caution. Patient referral patterns may influence local experience of this condition, and series reported from office practices tend to suggest a more favourable prognosis than cases reported from hospital and tertiary centres.[41–48]

Factors affecting metastatic potential of cutaneous squamous cell carcinoma (SCC)

Site

Tumour location influences prognosis: sites are listed in order of increasing metastatic potential.[30,41,49–52]

1 SCC arising at sun-exposed sites excluding lip and ear.
2 SCC of the lip.
3 SCC of the ear.
4 Tumours arising in non sun-exposed sites (e.g. perineum, sacrum, sole of foot).
5 SCC arising in areas of radiation or thermal injury, chronic draining sinuses, chronic ulcers, chronic inflammation or Bowen's disease.

Size: diameter

Tumours greater than 2 cm in diameter are twice as likely to recur locally (15.2% vs. 7.4%), and three times as likely to metastasize (30.3% vs. 9.1%) as smaller tumours.[41]

Size: depth

Tumours greater than 4 mm in depth (excluding surface layers of keratin) or extending down to the subcutaneous tissue (Clark level V) are more likely to recur and metastasize (metastatic rate 45.7%) compared with thinner tumours.[29,35,41] Recurrence and metastases are less likely in tumours confined to the upper half of the dermis and less than 4 mm in depth (metastatic rate 6.7%).[31,32,35,41]

Histological differentiation

Poorly differentiated tumours (i.e. those of Broders' grades 3 and 4; Appendix 2) have a poorer prognosis, with more than double the local recurrence rate and triple the metastatic rate of better differentiated SCC.[33,34,41] Tumours with perineural involvement are more likely to recur and to metastasize.[39,53] It seems logical that lymphatic or vascular invasion might imply a poor prognosis, but there is no evidence to support this as an independent risk factor.

Host immunosuppression

Tumours arising in patients who are immunosuppressed have a poorer prognosis. Host cellular immune response may be important both in determining the local invasiveness of

SCC and the host's response to metastases.[22,23,28]

Previous treatment and treatment modality

The risk of local recurrence depends upon the treatment modality. Locally recurrent disease itself is a risk factor for metastatic disease. Local recurrence rates are considerably less with Mohs' micrographic surgery than with any other treatment modality.[41,50–52,54,55]

Treatment

In interpreting and applying guidelines for treatment of SCC, three important points should be noted:

- There is a lack of randomized controlled trials (RCTs) for the treatment of primary cutaneous SCC.
- There is widely varying malignant behaviour of tumours which fall within the histological diagnostic category of 'primary cutaneous SCC'.
- There are varied experiences among the different specialists treating these tumours; these are determined by referral patterns and interests. Plastic and maxillofacial surgeons may encounter predominantly high-risk, aggressive tumours, whereas dermatologists may deal predominantly with smaller and less aggressive lesions.

However, there are three main factors which influence treatment, which are:

- the need for complete removal or treatment of the primary tumour;

- the possible presence of local 'in transit' metastases;
- the tendency of metastases to spread by lymphatics to lymph nodes.

The majority of SCCs are low risk and amenable to various forms of treatment, but it is essential to identify the significant proportion which are high-risk. These may be best managed by a multiprofessional team with experience of treating the most malignant tumours.[42,43,45,48,56–59]

The goal of treatment is complete (preferably histologically confirmed) removal or destruction of the primary tumour and of any metastases. In order to achieve this the margins of the tumour must be identified. The gold standard for identification of tumour margins is histological assessment, but most treatments rely on clinical judgement. It must be recognized that this is not always an accurate predictor of tumour extent, particularly when the margins of the tumour are ill-defined.[40,60–63]

SCC may give rise to local metastases, which are discontinuous with the primary tumour. Such 'in-transit' metastases may be removed by wide surgical excision or destroyed by irradiation of a wide field around the primary lesion. Small margins may not remove metastases in the vicinity of the primary tumour. Locally recurrent tumour may arise either due to failure to treat the primary continuous body of tumour, or from local metastases.[28,32,42,43,45,54,57,64,65]

SCC usually spreads to local lymph nodes and clinically enlarged nodes should be examined histologically (for example by fine needle aspiration or excisional biopsy). Tumour-positive lymph nodes are usually managed by regional node dissection, but detailed discussion of the management of metastatic disease is beyond the scope of these guidelines.[49,66–69]

In the absence of clinically enlarged nodes, techniques such as high resolution ultrasound-guided fine needle aspiration cytology may be useful in evaluating regional lymph nodes in patients with high risk tumours.[70–73] The role of sentinel lymph node biopsy has not been established.

Although there are many large series in which long-term outcome after treatment for cutaneous SCC has been reported (comprehensively summarized in reference 41), there are no large prospective randomized studies in which different treatments for this tumour have been compared.[42,63,74–76]

Guidelines for patient treatment

Conclusions from population-based studies do not necessarily indicate the best treatment for an individual patient. In particular, when choosing a treatment modality it is important to be aware of factors which may influence success. Curettage and cautery, cryosurgery, and to a lesser degree radiotherapy, are all techniques in which the outcome depends of the experience of the physician. Although the same could be said of surgical excision and Mohs' micrographic surgery, these two modalities provide tissue for histological examination which allows the pathologist to assess the adequacy of treatment and for the physician to undertake further surgery if necessary. For this reason, where feasible, surgical excision (including Mohs' micrographic surgery where appropriate) should be regarded as the treatment of first choice for cutaneous SCC. The other techniques can yield excellent results in experienced hands, but the quality of treatment cannot be assured or audited contemporaneously by a third party.[28,41,46,61,62,67,69,74,77–79]

Surgical excision

Surgical excision is the treatment of choice for the majority of cutaneous SCC. It allows full characterization of the tumour and a guide to the adequacy of treatment through histological examination of the margins of the excised tissue.[32,41]

When undertaking surgical excision a margin of normal skin is excised from around the tumour. For clinically well-defined, low risk tumours less than 2 cm in diameter, surgical excision with a minimum 4-mm margin around the tumour border is appropriate and would be expected to completely remove the primary tumour mass in 95% of cases[61] (*Strength of Recommendation A, Quality of Evidence II–iii*). Narrower margins of excision are more likely to leave residual tumour. In order to maintain the same degree of confidence of adequate excision, larger tumours, high risk tumours of Broders' grade 2, 3 or 4, tumours extending into the subcutaneous tissue and those in high-risk locations (ear, lip, scalp, eyelids, nose) should be removed with a wider margin (6 mm or more) and the tissue margins examined histologically, or with Mohs' micrographic surgery.[50–52,61]

It is only meaningful to consider such margins when the peripheral boundary of the tumour appears clinically well-defined. The concept of a 'surgical margin' (i.e. normal-appearing tissue around the tumour) is based upon an assumption that the clinically visible margin of the tumour bears a predictable relationship to the true extent of the tumour, and that excision of a margin of clinically normal-appearing tissue around the tumour will encompass any microscopic tumour extension. The wider the surgical margin the greater the likelihood that all tumour will be removed. Large tumours have greater microscopic tumour extension and should be removed with a wider margin. This concept is equally valid for non-surgical treatments such as radiotherapy and cryotherapy in which a margin of clinically normal-appearing tissue is treated around the tumour. Mohs' micrographic surgery does not make this assumption but displays the margins of the tissue for histological examination, and allows a primary tumour mass, growing in-continuity to be excised completely with minimal loss of normal tissue. There are important lessons to be learned from the experiences of micrographic surgery in treating cutaneous SCC (see below).[40,41,50–52,54,62]

Local metastases

Microscopic metastases may be found around high-risk primary cutaneous SCC.[43,65,68] Under these circumstances a 'wide' surgical margin extending well beyond the primary tumour may include such metastases and thus have a higher cure rate than a narrower margin. Mohs' micrographic surgery removes tumour growing in-continuity but does not identify in-transit micro-metastases. For this reason some practitioners of Mohs' micrographic surgery will excise a further surgical margin after the Mohs' surgical wound has been histologically confirmed to be clear of the primary tumour mass when treating high risk tumours.[43,68]

Histological assessment of surgical margins

Conventional histological examination of one or more transverse sections of excised tissue displays a cross-section of the tumour and tissue margins. This is the best way of assessing and categorizing the nature of the tumour, and it is usual to comment on whether the tumour

extends to the tissue margin, or if not, to record the margin of uninvolved skin around the tumour.[40] The value of such comments depends on how closely the section examined reflects the excised tissue in general. If SCC appears to extend to the margin of the examined tissue, then it should be assumed, particularly if the true margin of the tissue has been stained prior to sectioning, that excision is incomplete. Orientating markers or sutures should be placed in the surgical specimen by the surgeon to allow the pathologist to accurately report on the location of any residual tumour. A pathologist, using the conventional 'breadloaf' technique for examining tissue, typically views only a small sample of the specimen microscopically,[40] and this may allow incompletely excised high-risk tumour to go undetected. There are several alternative tissue preparations that allow the peripheral margins of the excised tissue to be more comprehensively examined.[60] The clinician and pathologist must work closely together in order to ensure appropriate sampling and microscopic examination of excised tissue, particularly with high-risk tumours.[40,60]

Mohs' micrographic surgery differs because the tissue is not displayed in cross-section and, if the first level of excision is adequate, tumour may not be seen at all in the microscopic sections. There are technical factors that may occasionally hamper identification of SCC in frozen sections and under these circumstances final histological examination should be undertaken on formalin-fixed tissue.[80,81]

Mohs' micrographic surgery

Mohs' micrographic surgery allows precise definition and excision of primary tumour growing in-continuity, and as such would be expected to reduce errors in primary treatment which may arise due to clinically invisible tumour extension. There is good evidence that the incidence of local recurrent and metastatic disease are low after Mohs' micrographic surgery and it should therefore be considered in the surgical treatment of high-risk SCC, particularly at difficult sites where wide surgical margins may be technically difficult to achieve without functional impairment[32,41] (*Strength of Recommendation B, Quality of Evidence II–iii*). The best cure rates for high risk SCCs are reported in series treated by Mohs' micrographic surgery.[41] Where Mohs' micrographic surgery is indicated but not available then one of the other histological techniques to examine the peripheral margin of the excised tissue should be employed.[60]

However, there are no prospective randomized studies comparing therapeutic outcome between conventional or wide surgical excision versus Mohs' micrographic surgery for cutaneous SCC.

It is firmly established that incomplete surgical excision is associated with a worse prognosis and, when doubt exists as to the adequacy of excision at the time of surgery, it is desirable, where practical, to delay or modify wound repair until complete tumour removal has been confirmed histologically.[28,41–45,53]

Curettage and cautery

Excellent cure rates have been reported in several series[41,63,74,78] and experience suggests that small (< 1 cm) well-differentiated, primary, slow-growing tumours arising on sun-exposed sites can be removed by experienced physicians with curettage. There are little published data relating outcome after curettage of larger tumours and different clinical tumour types.

The high cure rates reported following curettage and cautery of cutaneous SCC (*Quality of Evidence II–iii*) may reflect case selection, with a greater proportion of small tumours treated by curettage than by other techniques, but also raise the question as to whether curettage per se has a therapeutic advantage. The experienced clinician undertaking curettage can detect tumour tissue by its soft consistency and this may be of benefit in identifying invisible tumour extension and ensuring adequate treatment. Conventionally, cautery or electrodesiccation is applied to the curetted wound and the curettage–cautery cycle then repeated once or twice. In principle, curettage could be combined with other treatments such as surgical excision, cryotherapy or radiotherapy; it is routinely undertaken to 'debulk' the tumour prior to Mohs' micrographic surgery. Curettage provides poorly orientated material for histological examination and no histological assessment of the adequacy of treatment is possible. Curettage and cautery is not appropriate treatment for locally recurrent disease.

Cryosurgery

Good short term cure rates have been reported for small histologically confirmed SCC treated by cryosurgery in experienced hands. Prior biopsy is necessary to establish the diagnosis histologically. There is great variability in the use of liquid nitrogen for cryotherapy and significant transatlantic variations in practice. For this reason caution should be exercised in the use of cryotherapy for SCC, although it may be an appropriate technique for selected cases in specialized centres.[41,77] Cryosurgery is not appropriate for locally recurrent disease.

Radiotherapy

Radiation therapy alone offers reported short- and long-term cure rates for SCC which are comparable with other treatments.[32,41,74] Radiotherapy will, in certain circumstances, give the best cosmetic and/or functional result. This will often be the case for lesions arising on the lip, nasal vestibule, (and sometimes the outside of the nose) and ear, among others. Certain very advanced tumours, where surgical morbidity would be unacceptably high may also be best treated by radiotherapy.

Elective prophylactic lymph node dissection

Elective prophylactic lymph node dissection has been proposed for SCC on the lip greater than 6 mm in depth and cutaneous SCC greater than 8 mm in depth, but evidence for this is weak[46,49] (*Strength of Recommendation C, Quality of Evidence II–iii*). Elective lymph node dissection is not routinely practised and there is no compelling evidence of benefit over morbidity.[29,30,36]

The multiprofessional oncology team

Patients with high risk SCC and those presenting with clinically involved lymph nodes should ideally be reviewed by a multiprofessional oncology team which includes a dermatologist, pathologist, appropriately trained surgeon (usually a plastic or maxillofacial surgeon), clinical oncologist and a clinical nurse specialist in skin cancer. Some advanced tumours are not surgically respectable and these should be managed in a multiprofes-

Summary of treatment options for primary cutaneous squamous cell carcinoma

Treatment	Indications	Contraindications	Notes
Surgical excision	All resectable tumours	Where surgical morbidity is likely to be unreasonably high	Generally treatment of choice for SCC High risk tumours need wide margins or histological margin control
Mohs micrographic surgery/excision with histological control	High risk tumours, recurrent tumours	Where surgical morbidity is likely to be unreasonably high	Treatment of choice for high risk tumours
Radiotherapy	Non-resectable tumours	Where tumour margins are ill-defined	
Curettage and cautery	Small, well-defined low-risk tumours	High risk tumours	Curettage may be useful prior to surgical excision
Cryotherapy	Small, well-defined, low risk tumours	High risk tumours, recurrent tumours	Only suitable for experienced practitioners

sional setting in order that other therapeutic options are considered. Patients should be provided with suitable written information concerning diagnosis, prognosis and follow-up support, local and national support organizations and, where appropriate, access to a multiprofessional palliative care team.

Follow-up

Early detection and treatment improves survival of patients with recurrent disease. Ninety-five percent of local recurrences and 95% of metastases are detected within 5 years.[32,41] It would therefore seem reasonable for the patient who has had a high-risk SCC to be kept under observation for recurrent disease for this period of time (*Strength of Recommendation A, Quality of Evidence II–ii*). Patients should be, as far as possible, instructed in self-examination. Observation for recurrent disease may be undertaken by the specialist, primary care physician or by patient self-examination. The decision as to who follows the patient will depend upon the disease risk, local facilities and interests.[32,41]

References

1. Marks R. Squamous cell carcinoma. *Lancet* 1996; **347**: 735–8
2. Bernstein SC, Lim KK, Brodland DG, Heidelberg KA. The many faces of squamous cell carcinoma. *Dermatol Surg* 1996; **22**: 243–54
3. Glass AG, Hoover RN. The emerging epidemic of melanoma and squamous cell skin cancer. *JAMA* 1989; **262**: 2097–100
4. Gray DT, Suman VJ, Su WP *et al*. Trends in the population-based incidence of squamous cell carcinoma of the skin first diagnosed between 1984 and 1992. *Arch Dermatol* 1997; **133**: 735–40
5. Weinstock MA. The epidemic of squamous cell carcinoma. *JAMA* 1989; **262**: 2138–40
6. Baldursson B, Sigurgeirsson B, Lindelof B. Leg ulcers and squamous cell carcinoma. An epidemiological study and review of the literature. *Acta Derm Venereol* 1993; **73**: 171–4
7. Bosch RJ, Gallardo MA, Ruiz del Portal G *et al*. Squamous cell carcinoma secondary to recessive dystrophic epidermolysis bullosa: report of eight tumours in four patients. *J Eur Acad Dermatol Venereol* 1999; **13**: 198–204
8. Keefe M, Wakeel RA, Dick DC. Death from metastatic cutaneous squamous cell carcinoma in autosomal recessive dystrophic epidermolysis bullosa despite permanent inpatient care. *Dermatologica* 1988; **177**: 180–4
9. Chang A, Spencer JM, Kirsner RS. Squamous cell carcinoma arising from a nonhealing wound and osteomyelitis treated with Mohs' micrographic surgery: a case study. *Ostomy Wound Manage* 1998; **44**: 26–30
10. Chowdri NA, Darzi MA. Postburn scar carcinomas in Kashmiris. *Burns* 1996; **22**: 477–82
11. Dabski K, Stoll HL Jr, Milgrom H. Squamous cell carcinoma complicating late chronic discoid lupus erythematosus. *J Surg Oncol* 1986; **32**: 233–7
12. Fasching MC, Meland NB, Woods JE, Wolff BG. Recurrent squamous cell carcinoma arising in pilonidal sinus tract – multiple flap reconstructions. Report of a case. *Dis Colon Rectum* 1989; **32**: 153–8
13. Lister RK, Black MM, Calonje E, Burnand KG. Squamous cell carcinoma arising in chronic lymphoedema. *Br J Dermatol* 1997; **136**: 384–7
14. Maloney ME. Arsenic in dermatology. *Dermatol Surg* 1996; **22**: 301–4
15. Moy R, Eliezri YD. Significance of human

papilloma-induced squamous cell carcinoma to dermatologists. *Arch Dermatol* 1994; **130**: 235–8

16. Bens G, Wieland U, Hofmann A *et al.* Detection of new human papillomavirus sequences in skin lesions of a renal transplant recipient and characterization of one complete genome related to epidermodysplasia verruciformis-associated types. *J Gen Virol* 1998; **79**: 779–87

17. Harwood CA, McGregor JM, Proby CM, Breuer J. Human papillomavirus and the development of non-melanoma skin cancer. *J Clin Pathol* 1999; **52**: 249–53

18. Harwood CA, Surentheran T, McGregor JM *et al.* Human papillomavirus infection and non-melanoma skin cancer in immunosuppressed and immunocompetent individuals. *J Med Virol* 2000; **61**: 289–97

19. Glover MT, Niranjan N, Kwan JT, Leigh IM. Non-melanoma skin cancer in renal transplant recipients: the extent of the problem and a strategy for management. *Br J Plast Surg* 1994; **47**: 86–9

20. Liddington M, Richardson AJ, Higgins RM *et al.* Skin cancer in renal transplant recipients. *Br J Surg* 1989; **76**: 1002–5

21. Ong CS, Keogh AM, Kossard S *et al.* Skin cancer in Australian heart transplant recipients. *J Am Acad Dermatol* 1999; **40**: 27–34

22. Veness MJ, Quinn DI, Ong CS *et al.* Aggressive cutaneous malignancies following cardiothoracic transplantation: the Australian experience. *Cancer* 1999; **85**: 1758–64

23. Weimar VM, Ceilley RI, Goeken JA. Aggressive biologic behaviour of basal and squamous cell cancers in patients with chronic lymphocytic leukaemia or chronic lymphocytic lymphoma. *J Dermatol Surg Oncol* 1979; **5**: 609–14

24. Green A, Williams G, Neale R *et al.* Daily sunscreen application and betacarotene supplementation in prevention of basal-cell and squamous-cell carcinomas of the skin: a randomised controlled trial. *Lancet* 1999; **354**: 723–9

25. Marks R, Rennie G, Selwood TS. Malignant transformation of solar keratoses to squamous cell carcinoma in the skin: a prospective study. *Lancet* 1988; **9**: 795–7

26. Naylor MF, Boyd A, Smith DW *et al.* High sun protection factor sunscreens in the suppression of actinic neoplasia. *Arch Dermatol* 1995; **131**: 170–5

27. Thompson SC, Jolley D, Marks R. Reduction of solar keratosis by regular sunscreen use. *N Eng J Med* 1993; **329**: 1147–51

28. Barksdale SK, O'Connor N, Barnhill R. Prognostic factors for cutaneous squamous cell and basal cell carcinoma. Determinants of risk of recurrence, metastasis and development of subsequent skin cancers. *Surg Oncol Clin N Am* 1997; **6**: 625–38

29. Breuninger H, Black B, Rassner G. Microstaging of squamous cell carcinomas. *Am J Clin Pathol* 1990; **94**: 624–7

30. Breuninger H, Hawlitschek E. Das Mikrostaging des Plattenepithelkarzinoms der Haut und Lippen – lichtmikroskopisch erfasste Pronosenfaktoren. In: *Fortschritte der operativen und onkologischen Dermatologie* (Tilgen W, Petzoldt D, eds). Berlin, Heidelberg, New York: Springer, 1995; 110–15

31. Breuninger H, Langer B, Rassner G. Untersuchungen zur Prognosebestimmung des spinozellularen karzinoms der Haut und Unterlippe anhand des TNM-Systems und zusatzlicher Parameter. *Hautarzt* 1988; **39**: 430–4

32. Breuninger H. Diagnostic and therapeutic standards in interdisciplinary dermatologic oncology. German Cancer Society, 1998

33. Broders AC. Squamous cell epithelioma of the lip. *JAMA* 1920; **74**: 656–64

34. Broders AC. Squamous cell epithelioma of the skin. *Ann Surg* 1921; **73**: 141–60

35. Friedman HI, Cooper PH, Wanebo HJ. Prognostic and therapeutic use of microstaging in cutaneous squamous cell carcinoma of the trunk and extremities. *Cancer* 1985; **56**: 1099–105

36. Frierson HF, Cooper PH. Prognostic factors in squamous cell carcinoma of the lower lip. *Hum Pathol* 1986; **17**: 346–54

37. Heenan PJ, Elder DJ, Sobin LH. WHO international histological classification of tumors. Berlin, Heidelberg, New York: Springer, 1993

38. Hermanek P, Heuson DE, Hutter RVP, Sobin LH. UICC (International Union Against Cancer) TNM Supplement. Berlin, Heidelberg, New York: Springer, 1993

39. Mendenhall WM, Parsons JT, Mendenhall NP *et al*. Carcinoma of the skin of the head and neck with perineural invasion. *Head Neck* 1989; **11**: 301–8

40. Abide JM, Nahai F, Bennett RG. The meaning of surgical margins. *Plast Reconstr Surg* 1984; **73**: 492–6

41. Rowe DE, Carroll RJ, Day CL. Prognostic factors for local recurrence, metastasis and survival rates in squamous cell carcinoma of the skin, ear and lip. *J Am Acad Dermatol* 1992; **26**: 976–90

42. Dzubow LM, Rigel DS, Robins P. Risk factors for local recurrence of primary cutaneous squamous cell carcinomas. *Arch Dermatol* 1982; **118**: 900–2

43. Epstein E, Epstein NN, Bragg K, Linden G . Metastases from squamous cell carcinomas of the skin. *Arch Dermatol* 1968; **97**: 245–51

44. Epstein E. Malignant sun-induced squamous cell carcinoma of the skin. *J Dermatol Surg Oncol* 1983; **9**: 505–6

45. Eroglu A, Berberoglu U, Berberoglu S. Risk factors related to locoregional recurrence in squamous cell carcinoma of the skin. *J Surg Oncol* 1996; **61**: 124–30

46. Friedman NR. Prognostic factors for local recurrence, metastases and survival rates in squamous cell carcinoma of the skin, ear and lip. *J Am Acad Dermatol* 1993; **28**: 281–2

47. Katz AD, Urbach F, Lilienfeld AM. The frequency and risk of metastases in squamous cell carcinoma of the skin. *Cancer* 1957; **10**: 1162–6

48. Kwa RE, Campana K, Moy RL. Biology of cutaneous squamous cell carcinoma. *J Am Acad Dermatol* 1992; **26**: 1–26

49. Afzelius LE, Gunnarsson M, Nordgren H. Guidelines for prophylactic radical lymph node dissection in cases of carcinoma of the external ear. *Head Neck Surg* 1980; **2**: 361–5

50. Mohs FE, Snow SN. Microscopically controlled surgical treatment for squamous cell carcinoma of the lower lip. *Surg Gynecol Obstet* 1985; **160**: 37–41

51. Mohs FE. Chemosurgical treatment of cancer of the ear: a microscopically controlled method of excision. *Surgery* 1947; **21**: 605–22

52. Mohs FE. Chemosurgical treatment of cancer of the lip. *Arch Surg* 1944; **48**: 478–88

53. Cottel WI. Perineural invasion by squamous cell carcinoma. *J Dermatol Surg Oncol* 1982; **8**: 589–600

54. Glass RL, Spratt JS, Perez-Mesa C. The fate of inadequately excised epidermoid carcinoma of the skin. *Surg Gynecol Obstet* 1966; **122**: 245–8

55. Mohs FE. Chemosurgery. *Clin Plast Surg* 1980; **7**: 349–60

56. Immerman SC, Scanlon EF, Christ M, Knox KL. Recurrent squamous cell carcinoma of the skin. *Cancer* 1983; **51**: 1537–40

57. Kraus DH, Carew JF, Harrison LB. Regional lymph node metastasis from cutaneous squamous cell carcinoma. *Arch Otolaryngol Head Neck Surg* 1998; **124**: 582–7

58. Petter G, Haustein UF. Histologic subtyping and malignancy assessment of cutaneous squamous cell carcinoma. *Dermatol Surg* 2000; **26**: 521–30

59. Tavin E, Persky M. Metastatic cutaneous squamous cell carcinoma of the head and neck region. *Laryngoscope* 1996; **106**: 156–8

60. Rapini RP. Comparison of methods for checking surgical margins. *J Am Acad Dermatol* 1990; **23**: 288–94

61. Brodland DG, Zitelli JA. Surgical margins for excision of primary cutaneous squamous cell carcinoma. *J Am Acad Dermatol* 1992; **27**: 241–8

62. Fleming ID, Amonette R, Monaghan T, Fleming MD. Principles of management of basal and squamous cell carcinoma of the skin. *Cancer* 1995; **75**: 699–704

63. Knox JM, Freeman RG, Duncan WC, Heaton CL. Treatment of skin cancer. *Southern Med J* 1967; **60**: 241–6

64. Lund HZ. Metastasis from sun-induced squamous cell carcinoma of the skin: an uncommon event. *J Dermatol Surg Oncol* 1984; **10**: 169–70

65. Dinehart SM, Pollack SV. Metastases from squamous cell carcinoma of the skin and lip. *J Am Acad Dermatol* 1989; **21**: 241–8

66. Nicolson GL. Organ specificity of tumor metastasis: role of preferential adhesion, invasion and growth of malignant cells at specific secondary sites. *Cancer Metastasis Rev* 1988; **7**: 143–88

67. Weisberg NK, Bertagnolli MM, Becker DS. Combined sentinel lymphadenectomy and Mohs' micrographic surgery for high-risk cutaneous squamous cell carcinoma. *J Am Acad Dermatol* 2000; **43**: 483–8

68. Brodland DG, Zitelli JA. Mechanisms of metastasis. *J Am Acad Dermatol* 1992; **27**: 1–8

69. Geohas J, Roholt NS, Robinson JK. Adjuvant radiotherapy after excision of cutaneous squamous cell carcinoma. *J Am Acad Dermatol* 1994; **30**: 633–6

70. van den Brekel MWM, Stel HV, Castelijns JA et al. Lymph node staging in patients with clinically negative neck examinations by ultrasound and ultrasound-guided aspiration cytology. *Am J Surg* 1991; **162**: 362–6

71. Vassallo P, Wernecke K, Roos N, Peters PE. Differentiation of benign from malignant superficial lymphadenopathy: the role of high resolution US. *Radiology* 1992; **183**: 215–20

72. Knappe M, Louw M, Gregor RT. Ultrasonography-guided fine-needle aspiration for the assessment of cervical metastases. *Arch Otolaryngol Head Neck Surg* 2000; **126**: 1091–6

73. Sumi M, Ohki M, Nakamura T. Comparison of sonography and CT for differentiating benign from malignant cervical lymph nodes in patients with squamous cell carcinoma of the head and neck. *AJR Am J Roentgenol* 2001; **176**: 1019–24

74. Freeman RG, Knox JM, Heaton CL. The treatment of skin cancer. A statistical study of 1341 skin tumours comparing results obtained with irradiation, surgery and curettage followed by electrodesiccation. *Cancer* 1964; **17**: 535–8

75. Macomber WB, Wang MKH, Sullivan JG. Cutaneous epithelioma. *Plast Reconst Surgery* 1959; **24**: 545–62

76. Stenbeck KD, Balanda KP, Williams MJ et al. Patterns of treated non-melanoma skin cancer in Queensland – the region with the highest incidence rates in the world. *Med J Aust* 1990; **153**: 511–15

77. Kuflik EG, Gage AA. The five-year cure rate achieved by cryosurgery for skin cancer. *J Am Acad Dermatol* 1991; **24**: 1002–4

78. Tromovitch TA. Skin cancer. Treatment by curettage and desiccation. *Calif Med* 1965; **103**: 107–8

79. Karagas MR. Occurrence of cutaneous basal cell and squamous cell malignancies among those with a prior history of skin cancer. *J Invest Dermatol* 1994; **102**: 10–13S

80. Telfer NR. Mohs' micrographic surgery for cutaneous squamous cell carcinoma: practical considerations. *Br J Dermatol* 2000; **142**: 631–3

81. Turner RJ, Leonard N, Malcolm AJ et al. A retrospective study of outcome of Mohs' micrographic surgery for cutaneous squamous cell carcinoma using formalin fixed sections. *Br J Dermatol* 2000; **142**: 752–7

82. Griffiths CEM. The British Association of Dermatologists guidelines for the management of skin disease. *Br J Dermatol* 1999; **141**: 396–7

Appendix 1

Full details of the British Association of Dermatologists' guidelines process are published in a previous edition of the journal.[82]

Strength of recommendations

A   There is good evidence to support the use of the procedure.

B   There is fair evidence to support the use of the procedure.

C   There is poor evidence to support the use of the procedure.

D   There is fair evidence to support the rejection of the use of the procedure.

E   There is good evidence to support the rejection of the use of the procedure.

Quality of evidence

I   Evidence obtained from at least one properly designed, randomized control trial.

II–I   Evidence obtained from well designed controlled trials without randomization.

II–ii   Evidence obtained from well designed cohort or case control analytic studies, preferably from more than one centre or research group.

II–iii   Evidence obtained from multiple time series with or without the intervention. Dramatic results in uncontrolled experiments (such as the introduction of penicillin treatment in the 1940s) could also be regarded as this type of evidence.

III   Opinions of respected authorities based on clinical experience, descriptive studies or reports of expert committees.

IV   Evidence inadequate owing to problems of methodology (e.g. sample size, or length or comprehensiveness of follow-up or conflicts in evidence).

Appendix 2

Broders' histological classification of differentiation in squamous cell carcinoma

Broders devised a classification system in which grades 1, 2 and 3 denoted ratios of differentiated to undifferentiated cells of 3:1, 1:1 and 1:3, respectively. Grade 4 denoted tumour cells having no tendency towards differentiation.

Appendix IV
U.K. guidelines for the management of cutaneous melanoma

DLL Roberts, AV Anstey, RJ Barlow and NH Cox on behalf of the British Association of Dermatologists, and JA Newton Bishop, PG Corrie, J Evans, ME Gore, PN Hall and N Kirkham on behalf of the Melanoma Study Group

Footnote

Contribution to these guidelines has been made by a large number of clinicians who are members of the Melanoma Study Group and the British Association of Dermatologists. They have also been endorsed by or have had input from representatives of the following groups or organizations: the Royal College of Physicians, London; the Royal College of Pathologists (pathology section only); the Department of Health; the British Association of Plastic Surgeons, London; the Royal College of Radiologists, London; the Specialty Advisory Board in Plastic Surgery of the Royal College of Surgeons of Edinburgh; the Royal College of Surgeons of England; the Royal College of General Practitioners, London.

Members of the British Association of Dermatologists Therapy Guidelines and Audit subcommittee are NH Cox (Chairman), AV Anstey, CB Bunker, MJDGoodfield, AS Highet, D Mehta, RH Meyrick Thomas and JK Schofield. The Multiprofessional Skin Cancer Committee representing the British Association of Dermatologists, the British Association of Plastic Surgeons and members of the Faculty of Clinical Oncology of the Royal College of Radiologists consisted of NH Cox (Chairman), AY Finlay, BR Allen, D Murray, RW Griffiths, A Batchelor, D Morgan, JK Schofield, CB Bunker, NR Telfer, GB Colver, PW Bowers and the authors.

Disclaimer

These guidelines reflect the best published data available at the time the report was prepared. Caution should be exercised in interpreting the data; the results of future studies may require alteration of the conclusions or recommendations in this report. It may be necessary or even desirable to depart from the guidelines in the interests of specific patients and special circumstances. Just as adherence to the guidelines may not constitute defence against a claim of negligence, so deviation from them should not be necessarily deemed negligent.

Summary

These guidelines for management of cutaneous melanoma present evidence-based guidance for treatment, with identification of the strength of evidence available at the time of preparation of the guidelines, and a brief overview of epidemiological aspects, diagnosis and investigation. To reflect the collaborative process for the U.K., they are subject to dual publication in the *British Journal of Dermatology* and the *British Journal of Plastic Surgery*.

These consensus guidelines have been drawn up by a multidisciplinary working party with membership drawn from a variety of groups and co-ordinated by the Melanoma Study Group and the British Association of Dermatologists. The guidelines deal with aspects of the management of melanoma from the prevention of melanoma through the stages of diagnosis and initial treatment to palliation of advanced disease. Levels of evidence to support the guidelines are quoted according to the criteria stated in Table 1. The consultation process for British Association of Dermatologists guidelines has been published elsewhere.[1] Where no level is quoted the evidence is to be regarded as representing level IV (i.e. a consensus statement). The intention of the working party was to come to a consensus about current best practice for the management of this type of cancer in the belief that the development of such a consensus will promote good standards of care across the whole country. The guidelines are, however, guidelines only. Care should be individualized wherever appropriate.

The guidelines are also intended to promote the integration of care between medical and paramedical specialties for the benefit of the patient. Multidisciplinary care of the patient is held to be the most desirable model as recommended in the report of Calman and Hine.[2] The guidelines document is concerned with a national consensus but it is hoped that it will assist regional groups in defining local policies.

Caution should be exercised in interpreting the data; the results of future studies may require alteration of the conclusions or recommendations in this report. Possible audit points for melanoma are given in Appendix 1. These guidelines are planned to be updated in 2003.

Prevention of melanoma

Individuals, and particularly children, should not get sunburnt (level III).[3,4] White-skinned individuals should limit their total cumulative sun exposure through life.[5,6] Lesions that are not obviously benign, or changing moles, should be seen by family doctors and either removed in their entirety for pathological examination, or referred and dealt with by appropriately trained specialists (level III).

Clinical diagnosis of melanoma

The seven-point checklist emphasizing a history of change in size, shape and colour of a pre-existing pigmented lesion is recommended for use for both patient and general practitioner education.[7]

Major features are:

- change in size;
- irregular shape;
- irregular colour.

Minor features are:

- largest diameter 7 mm or more;
- inflammation;
- oozing;
- change in sensation.

Lesions with any of the major features or three minor ones are suspicious of melanoma.[8] Suspicious lesions should ideally be seen by specialists, that is clinicians routinely treating large numbers of patients with pigmented lesions. Where suspicious lesions are biopsied they should be removed completely and sent for histopathological examination.

Referral

Early recognition of malignant melanoma presents the best opportunity for cure. It is therefore incumbent on dermatologists to provide a service that allows rapid access for diagnosis and management, particularly in view of the Government's suggestion that patients with potential malignant melanoma should be seen within 2 weeks of receipt of a referral letter from the general practitioner. Clearly identified 'pigmented lesion clinics' have been shown to be an effective means of providing rapid access to expert medical services for patients with pigmented lesions, although they may have little impact on melanoma mortality at a population level.[9,10]

Recommendations for referral

- Patients with lesions suspicious of melanoma should be referred urgently to a

dermatologist or surgeon/plastic surgeon with an interest in pigmented lesions.
- These specialists should ensure that a system is in place to enable patients with suspicious lesions to be seen within 2 weeks of receipt of the referral letter.
- All patients who have had lesions removed by their general practitioner that are subsequently reported as melanoma should be referred immediately to specialists.

(Grade C, level III)

Initial assessment and management

Any patient with a pigmented lesion that the specialist feels is clinically suspicious of melanoma should have a full skin examination. The site and size of the pigmented lesion should be documented and a record should be made of other pigmented lesions. Clinical photographs may be helpful. The patient should be carefully examined for lymphadenopathy and hepatomegaly.

Recommendations for record keeping of clinical features

As a minimum the following should be included:

- History (the presence or absence of these changes should be recorded):
  Change in size
  Change in colour
  Change in shape
  Symptoms (itching, bleeding etc.)

- Examination
    Site
    Size
    Description (noting irregular margins, irregular pigmentation and ulceration if present)
    Other pigmented lesions
    Any regional lymphadenopathy
    Examination for hepatomegaly
                                    (Grade B, level III)

Screening and surveillance of high-risk individuals

Primary care teams, as well as cancer units and centres, have a responsibility to raise public awareness of skin cancer. The incidence of melanoma in the U.K. is approximately 10 cases per 100,000 per annum.[11–13]

There are some individuals at higher risk of melanoma who should be considered for referral to specialist clinics. These individuals can be divided broadly into two groups based upon the degree of risk.

1. Individuals at moderate increased risk (approximately 8–10 times that of the general population) should be counselled about this risk and taught how to self-examine for changing naevi, but very long-term follow-up is not usual. Such patients are those with either a previous primary melanoma,[14] or large numbers of moles, some of which are clinically atypical.[15,16]
2. Those at greatly increased risk of melanoma (at least 100 times that of the general population). Patients with a giant congenital pigmented hairy naevus[17,18] (definitions include: '20 cm or more in diameter' and '5% of body surface area') should be monitored by an expert for their life time because of the risk of malignant change,

which is significant but poorly quantified. Excision biopsy of suspicious areas in large congenital naevi may be necessary but requires expert histopathological review. By contrast, surgical excision of small congenital naevi is not considered necessary in the absence of suspicious features.

Patients with a strong family history of melanoma are also at greatly increased risk. Those with three or more cases of melanoma in the extended family should be referred to appropriate clinics managing inherited predisposition to cancer (involving dermatologists and/or clinical geneticists) for counselling. It is the consensus of the Melanoma Genetics Consortium that it is premature to suggest gene testing but this may change as more is known of the genes predisposing to melanoma.[19] The risk associated with the presence of two family members affected with melanoma is lower. In these families, if affected individuals also have the atypical mole syndrome, or if there is a history of multiple primary tumours in an individual, then referral should also be made for counselling; otherwise, family members should probably be considered at moderately increased risk.

This group of particularly high-risk individuals should be advised on the specific changes that suggest melanoma and encouraged to undertake monthly self-examination (level III). Photography may be a useful adjunct to detecting early melanoma in either of these high-risk groups (level III).

Recommendations for screening and surveillance of high-risk individuals

- Patients who have already had a melanoma or who have the atypical mole syndrome are at moderately increased risk of another primary, and should be advised of this and taught how to recognize a melanoma.

- Patients with giant congenital pigmented naevi are at increased risk of melanoma and require long-term follow-up.
- The prophylactic excision of small congenital naevi is not recommended.
- Individuals with a family history of three or more cases of melanoma should be referred to a Department of Clinical Genetics for counselling. Those with two cases in the family may also benefit, especially if one of the cases had multiple primary melanomas or the atypical mole syndrome.

(Grade B, level IIa)

Biopsy of suspected melanoma

Excision of a lesion suspected to be melanoma should be performed as a full-thickness skin biopsy to include the whole tumour with a 2–5-mm clinical margin of normal skin later-ally and with a cuff of subdermal fat. This allows confirmation of the diagnosis, such that subsequent definitive treatment can be based on Breslow thickness.

Shave and punch biopsies are not recom-mended because they will at the very least make the pathological staging of the lesion impossible (level III). Incisional biopsy is occasionally acceptable, for example in the differential diagnosis of lentigo maligna on the face or of acral melanoma, but there is no place for incisional biopsy in primary care (level III). There is little evidence that incisional biopsies of melanoma affect the prognosis[20,21] although one paper suggests that there may be an adverse effect in lesions situated on the head and neck.[22]

Biopsies of possible subungual melanomas should be carried out by surgeons regularly doing so. The nail should be removed and clinically obvious tumour or, in the absence of a mass, the nail matrix should be adequately sampled.

Prophylactic excision of pigmented lesions or of small congenital naevi in the absence of suspicious features is futile and not to be recommended.

Histopathology

Recommendations for the reporting of tissues removed as part of the surgical treatment of cutaneous melanoma have been published in an international consensus statement supple-mented by a proposed final revised staging system for cutaneous melanoma published recently.[23] Table 2 gives the recommended American Joint Committee on Cancer staging system.

Pathology request forms must be accurately completed and give full identification details. The whole lesion should be adequately sampled, probably by serial transverse slicing of the biopsy at approximately 2-mm inter-vals, processing all of the slices and examining sections cut at three levels. The pathologist's report should include the following minimum data:

- The site of the tumour.
- The type of surgical procedure: excision or re-excision, incision biopsy, punch biopsy, shave biopsy, curettage, other.
- A full description of the macroscopic

appearance of the tumour, and the dimensions of the specimen in millimetres.

- When possible, a statement of whether the lesion is primary, locally recurrent or metastatic to the site.
- Whether there is ulceration.
- The Breslow thickness of the tumour, measured from the granular layer of the epidermis to the base of the tumour, to the nearest 0.1 mm. Ulcerated tumours should be measured from the base of the ulcer to the base of the tumour. Tumour forming a sheath around appendages should be excluded when making measurements.
- The depth of penetration of the dermis (Clark's level) may also be stated, although this is a less reliable indicator of prognosis than Breslow thickness in most circumstances.
- The presence of radial growth phase tumour alone or vertical growth phase.
- The frequency of mitotic figures mm^{-2} (vertical growth phase only).
- The presence or absence of tumour regression.
- The presence (and, if present, the degree) or absence of a lymphocytic inflammatory infiltrate in, or in response to, the tumour (level II).
- The presence of any obvious lymphatic or vascular invasion or perineural invasion.
- The histogenetic type of melanoma, including the presence of desmoplasia and/or neurotropism.
- The presence of microsatellites.
- Whether excision is complete, and the minimum margin of excision to peripheral or deep surgical margin, measured in millimetres. If excision is not complete, the residual disease should be identified as *in situ* or invasive.
- Pathological staging (TNM) and coding (e.g. SNOMED code).

Definitive treatment of the primary lesion

Surgical excision margins for invasive melanoma depend on the Breslow thickness as measured by the histopathologist and are based on two randomized clinical trials[24,25] and a National Institutes of Health Consensus Panel.[26] The recommended surgical margins are those measured clinically at the time of surgery, rather than the histopathological margins measured microscopically. The margins suggested may need to be adjusted for cosmetic or functional reasons, for example around the eye.

Lentigo maligna

Initial incisional biopsy is appropriate for changing flat pigmented lesions on the face which may represent lentigo maligna, although sampling problems occasionally mean that biopsies may not be representative of the whole lesion.

Histologically confirmed lentigo maligna is best treated by complete excision because of the risk of invasive change. The risk of progression is, however, poorly established and in the very elderly may be unlikely within their life span. Therefore, for some particular clinical situations, treatment by other methods such as radiotherapy, cryotherapy or observation only[27-30] may be appropriate, although the risk of recurrence is higher than with surgery.[31-33] If the patient with lentigo maligna is treated by non-surgical means then the reason for this choice should be clearly documented.

Lentigo maligna and other *in situ* melanomas have no potential for metastatic spread and the aim should be to excise the lesion completely with a clear histological margin. No further treatment is then required. Local recurrence of other types of *in situ* melanoma is rare, but recurrence of lentigo maligna is common and is usually attributed to a 'field effect', whereby atypical melanocytes extend laterally along the epidermis but are not clinically detectable.[34]

Lesions less than 1 mm in depth

The recommended surgical margins are based on the World Health Organization Trial.[25] This randomized trial compared 1-cm and 3-cm margins for melanomas up to 2 mm thick. No local recurrences were seen in patients with melanomas less than 1 mm in depth with either excision margin, and a 1-cm margin was deemed safe and appropriate for these lesions. Thin tumours less than 0.75 mm in Breslow thickness without vertical growth phase are commonly excised with a 0.5-cm margin or even less.[35,36] It is the consensus view that this margin is probably adequate but there are no data to support this conclusion.

Lesions 1–2 mm in depth

There have been two large randomized studies that have included patients in this category. The World Health Organization Study[25] showed no difference in overall patient survival between 1-cm and 3-cm margins in this group. However, there were four patients who developed local recurrences as the first sign of relapse. All these patients had undergone 1-cm excision and each had a primary lesion between 1 and 2 mm thick. The authors were therefore cautious in recommending 1-cm margins for this group and suggested that 2-cm margins may be more appropriate until further follow-up is completed. It is recommended that the decision about margin should be made by the multidisciplinary team after discussion with the patient but that a 1-cm margin should be the minimum where functionally and cosmetically sensible. The Intergroup Melanoma Trial compared 2-cm vs. 4-cm margins of excision for lesions of 1–4 mm in depth.[24] No difference was seen between the two groups in either local recurrence or survival. Margins greater than 2 cm are therefore inappropriate in this group.

Recommended surgical excision margins

Breslow thickness	Excision margins	Approximate 5-year survival	Grading of evidence
In situ	2–5-mm clinical margins to achieve complete histological excision	95–100%[a]	Level B, grade III
Less than 1 mm	1 cm (narrower margins are probably safe in lesions less than 0.75 mm in depth)	95–100%	Level A, grade I
1–2 mm	1–2 cm	80–96%	Level A, grade I
2.1–4 mm	2–3 cm (2 cm preferred)	60–75%	Level A, grade I
Greater than 4 mm	2–3 cm	50%	Level B, grade III

[a]In theory recurrence should never occur after in situ melanoma, but occasional cases do recur.[38,39] The assumption is that regression at diagnosis obscured a more advanced tumour, or that progression occurred after incomplete removal of the in situ disease.

Lesions 2–4 mm in depth

On the basis of the Intergroup Melanoma Trial it has been shown that there is no difference between 2-cm and 4-cm margins for this group, in either overall survival or recurrence rates.[24] The results of a randomized trial comparing 1-cm with 3-cm margins are awaited. It seems reasonable to suggest, on the basis of published evidence, that 2-cm margins are safe and should be taken where possible.

Lesions greater than 4 mm in depth

Deeper tumours have not been included in any of the randomized studies. The local recurrence rate is high and metastatic spread is common. It would seem reasonable to suggest margins of 2 cm and that there is probably no advantage in margins over 3 cm, but data to confirm this are limited.[37]

Investigations for patients with melanoma

No investigations are necessary for patients with stage I disease. Stage I and IIA melanoma patients should not be staged by imaging, as the true-positive pick-up rate is low and the false-positive rate is high.[40,41]

Patients at intermediate or high risk of recurrent disease (stage IIB and over) should have the following staging investigations: chest X-ray; liver ultrasound or computed tomographic (CT) scan with contrast of chest, abdomen ± pelvis; liver-function tests/lactate dehydrogenase; and full blood count. In the absence of effective chemotherapy for melanoma, however, it may be reasonable to omit scanning in individual stage IIB patients. There is no place for a bone scan in staging except where symptoms point to possible bone disease.

Ideally, patients with stage IIB or more advanced melanoma should be managed in a Cancer Centre by a skin cancer multidisciplinary team, either *in toto* or as shared care with a Cancer Unit. This team should include a dermatologist, surgeon, oncologist, pathologist, radiologist, counsellor, specialist nurse and palliative care specialist. Communication with the primary health care team should be optimized.

Adjuvant therapy

There are no adjuvant therapies of proven benefit for melanoma as yet, but several clinical trials are actively recruiting patients. Patients at intermediate or high risk of relapse should be referred to the multidisciplinary team based at a Cancer Centre, staged (see investigations list above – these may vary according to study protocol) and considered for a trial of adjuvant therapy without delay (stages IIB, IIC or III). Most trials require entry within 8 weeks of completion of surgery and therefore this referral to the Cancer Centre should be prompt.

Patients should be offered entry into clinical trials wherever possible. This is particularly important in the context of adjuvant therapy. Clinicians involved in the care of patients with melanoma should regularly update themselves on the clinical trials available to their patients. This can be done through the local Cancer Centre or the Melanoma Group of the National Cancer Research Institute (Tel. 020 7269 3548). Entry criteria vary but, in general, those with stage IIB or stage III disease can be considered, although this may change with time.

There is currently no standard adjuvant systemic therapy for patients with melanoma. In the U.S.A., following the ECOG 1684 trial the 'Kirkwood' high-dose interferon regimen is regarded as standard therapy for patients at high risk of recurrence[42] although the ECOG 1690 trial was non-confirmatory.[43] A recent study comparing 1 year's treatment with high-dose interferon with a vaccine to gangliosides (anti-GM2) was closed after interim analysis because of apparent better survival of the interferon-treated group.[44] Further trials continue to be reported. Views on standard therapy may be modified in light of further information from other trials. Although interferon is now licensed for adjuvant use in the U.K., a second confirmatory trial with mature data is considered necessary before this regimen can be recommended as standard treatment, not least because of the side-effects commonly experienced. Adjuvant therapies should be delivered by specialists.

The role of vaccines as adjuvant therapies remains to be established.

There is no role for adjuvant isolated limb perfusion (ILP)[45] (level Ib), although it may have a role in preoperative reduction of tumour volume.

Recommendations for investigations and adjuvant therapy

* Stage I and IIA melanoma patients should not be staged by imaging as the true-positive pick-up rate is low and the false-positive rate is high. This recommendation would be revised if effective therapy for visceral melanoma were identified (grade A, level II).

* Stage IIB and over patients should be referred to a Cancer Centre service for consideration of trials of adjuvant therapies.

* The role of interferon as an adjuvant therapy remains to be established (grade C, level I).

Management of clinically node-negative patients

There is currently no place for elective lymph node dissection outside a clinical trial (grade A, level I).[46,47] Sentinel lymph node (SLN) biopsy was developed as a means of identifying the first lymph node draining the skin in which the melanoma arises.[48] The procedure is carried out at the same time as definitive (wider) excision of the primary tumour. Patients with a positive SLN proceed to excision of nodes in the relevant nodal basin. At the present time SLN biopsy appears to be useful for staging in clinical stage II melanoma, and can be used as part of the staging strategy in those centres that are skilled and experienced in the technique. The procedure is associated with some morbidity. Until there is further evidence that there is an improvement in prognosis as a result of use of this technique to identify patients in whom therapeutic lymph node dissection should be performed, SLN biopsy is not generally recommended for routine use, and preferably should only be performed as part of a clinical study or trial. This is an area where reports of on-going multicentre studies are anticipated and current recommendations may need to be reconsidered.

Recommendations for the management of clinically node-negative patients

- There is no role for elective lymph node dissection (grade E, level I).
- Sentinel node biopsy can be used for staging in stage II melanoma in specialist centres in clinical trials but unless evidence emerges for a role in determining outcome it should not be routine (grade C, level IIa).

Management of patients with clinically or radiologically suspicious lymph nodes

Fine needle aspiration cytology (FNAC) of nodes is recommended when there is clinical doubt about the significance of the nodes. This may need to be repeated if there is a negative result but on-going suspicion. Open biopsy is recommended when there is clinical suspicion even in the presence of negative FNACs in which lymphocytes have been successfully aspirated. If open biopsy is performed, the incision must be such as to allow subsequent complete formal block dissection of the regional nodes without compromise.

Management of patients with confirmed positive lymph node metastasis

Radical lymph node dissections should be performed by those with expertise in the surgery of this condition. Prior to block dissec-

tion, staging investigations should be carried out as listed previously. Imaging of the liver by either CT scan or ultrasound should be performed preoperatively. Where preoperative scanning would necessitate delay to surgery that is considered necessary even if widespread disease were to be detected, postoperative scanning may be carried out. The decision as to whether or not surgery should proceed prior to scanning should be made after careful discussion with an informed patient.

The management of regional lymph node metastases is as follows:

- If only one or two involved nodes are present below the inguinal ligament, a subinguinal node dissection of the femoral triangle is indicated.
- If there is gross involvement of the subinguinal nodes, or if the node of Cloquet is involved, then some would recommend extended dissection to include the iliac and obturator nodes to prevent local recurrence (level III).[49]
- Where relapse involves further lymph node basins, these should be treated by block dissection. In the neck, a functional dissection is ideally performed although in more locally advanced disease a radical neck dissection may be appropriate.
- A block dissection specimen should be marked and orientated for the pathologist. The pathologist should be asked to report on the number of nodes in the specimen and the presence of any extracapsular spread.

Locoregional recurrent melanoma: skin and soft tissues

Where possible in the case of single local or regional metastases, surgery is the treatment of choice. Patients with multiple local metastases in a limb should be referred to a centre specializing in regional therapy where the following may be considered: ILP or limb infusion with cytotoxic agents; and carbon dioxide laser ablation for multiple small superficial lesions (level III).[50] Radiotherapy is not recommended in the first instance (level III).

Recommendations for locoregional recurrent melanoma

- Nodes clinically suspicious of melanoma should be sampled using fine needle aspiration cytology (FNAC) prior to carrying out formal block dissection. If FNAC is negative although lymphocytes were seen, an open biopsy should be performed if suspicion remains (grade B, level III).
- Prior to formal dissection, performed by an expert, staging by scan should be carried out other than where this would mean unnecessary delay (grade B, level III).
- The treatment of locoregional recurrence in a limb is palliative. Initial treatment is usually surgical, followed, where necessary, by carbon dioxide laser treatment and possibly isolated limb perfusion (grade B, level II).

Occult primary melanoma

Patients with occult primary melanoma will present with lymph node disease, a single soft-tissue metastasis or systemic disease in the absence of a recognizable primary. The present-ing lymph nodes or systemic metastases should be treated appropriately regardless of the inability to detect the primary lesion (level III).

Metastatic disease

All patients should have access to a palliative care team providing expertise in symptom control and psychosocial support. Links should be made with community cancer support networks as soon as possible.

Consideration of surgical removal of localized metastases should be made (e.g. skin metastases, solitary brain metastases[51,52] and occasionally those in other sites). Radiotherapy to bone or skin metastases can provide short-term symptomatic control[53] and has a palliative value in patients with brain metastases.[54,55]

Patients with unresectable metastatic disease should be referred to a specialist oncologist for management advice. Standard chemotherapy outside a clinical trial remains single-agent dacarbazine[56] but no systemic therapy has yet been shown to prolong significantly the survival of patients with metastatic melanoma. Thus, these patients, wherever possible, should be considered for and then counselled about entry into clinical trials of novel therapies, in addition to being offered standard palliative measures.

Melanoma, hormone replacement therapy and pregnancy

There is no evidence that melanoma at or near the time of pregnancy adversely affects the prognosis, but the data are limited.[57,58] The Breslow thickness, site and presence of ulceration are still the key determinants (level III).

Advice about continuance of and future pregnancies should be given based on the patient's prognosis and the possible social consequences of it; that is, the relative chance that a mother might die when her child was young, compared with that of a woman of the same age without melanoma. These social or family considerations may also be relevant to a male patient whose partner is pregnant or if he and his partner are considering a pregnancy.

There is no conclusive evidence that either hormone replacement therapy or the use of the oral contraceptive pill play any role in the natural history of melanoma (level III).

Recommendations for metastatic disease, hormone replacement therapy and pregnancy

- Consideration of surgically resectable metastases should be made, such as in the skin, brain or gut (grade B, level II).
- Radiotherapy may have a palliative role in the treatment of metastases (grade B, level II).
- The standard chemotherapy of choice is dacarbazine although its role is palliative (grade C, level II).
- There are no data contraindicating the use of the contraceptive pill or hormone replacement therapy after melanoma (grade B, level II).
- The risk of subsequent pregnancy on outcome from melanoma is not known.

Follow-up

All patients should be taught self-examination because many recurrences are found by patients themselves at home rather than by clinicians in the clinic.

Patients with *in situ* melanoma need be reviewed only once after complete excision of the primary lesion.[59]

All patients with invasive melanoma should be followed up 3-monthly for 3 years. In stage I disease some view this frequency of follow-up as excessive; the decision about frequency may be made on an individual basis according to the need to monitor naevi and emotional state. Thereafter, patients with melanomas less than 1.0 mm in depth may be discharged from routine follow-up; other patients should be followed up for a further 2 years at 6-monthly intervals.[59]

The following should be examined and details recorded at each follow-up: site of primary and adjacent skin, for local recurrences and local metastatic disease; the draining lymph node basins, for lymphadenopathy; the remaining skin, for any other suspicious pigmented lesion. Regular radiological imaging is currently not a necessity but clinical photography may be helpful in follow-up, particularly in those with multiple atypical moles.

Recommendations for follow-up

- Patients with *in situ* melanomas do not require follow-up.
- Patients with invasive melanomas should be followed up 3-monthly for 3 years. Where the melanoma thickness was less

than 1 mm the patient may be discharged; others should be followed-up for a further 2 years at 6-monthly intervals. (Grade C)

References

1. Griffiths CEM. The British Association of Dermatologists guidelines for the management of skin disease. *Br J Dermatol* 1999; **141**: 396–7.
2. Calman K, Hine D. *Report by the Advisory Group on Cancer Services to the Chief Medical Officers of England and Wales.* Department of Health/Welsh Office, 1995.
3. Marks R, Whiteman D. Sunburn and melanoma: how strong is the evidence? *Br Med J* 1994; **308**: 75–6.
4. Whiteman D, Green A. Melanoma and sunburn. *Cancer Causes Control* 1994; **5**: 564–72.
5. Armstrong BK. Epidemiology of malignant melanoma: intermittent or total accumulated exposure to the sun? *J Dermatol Surg Oncol* 1988; **14**: 835–49.
6. Armstrong BK, Kricker A. Sun exposure causes both nonmelanocytic skin cancer and malignant melanoma. In: *Proceedings on Environmental UV Radiation and Health Effects*, 1993; 106–13.
7. MacKie RM. *Malignant Melanoma: a Guide to Early Diagnosis*, 1994.
8. Du Vivier AWP, Williams HC, Brett JV, Higgins EM. How do malignant melanomas present and does this correlate with the seven-point check-list? *Clin Exp Dermatol* 1991; **16**: 344–7.
9. Melia J, Cooper EJ, Frost T *et al.* Cancer Research Campaign health education programme to promote the early detection of cutaneous malignant melanoma. I. Work-load and referral patterns. *Br J Dermatol* 1995; **132**: 405–13.
10. Melia J. Early detection of cutaneous

11. MacKie RM, Hole D, Hunter JAA *et al.* Cutaneous malignant melanoma in Scotland: incidence, survival, and mortality, 1979–94. The Scottish Melanoma Group. *Br Med J* 1997; **315**: 1117–21.
12. Melia J. Changing incidence and mortality from cutaneous malignant melanoma. *Br Med J* 1997; **315**: 1106–7.
13. Parkin DM, Muir CS, Whelan SL *et al.* Cancer incidence in five continents: comparability and quality of data. *IARC Sci Publ* 1992; **120**: 45–173.
14. Rhodes AR, Weinstock MA, Fitzpatrick TB *et al.* Risk factors for cutaneous melanoma. A practical method of recognizing predisposed individuals. *JAMA* 1987; **258**: 3146–54.
15. Newton JA, Bataille V, Griffiths K *et al.* How common is the atypical mole syndrome phenotype in apparently sporadic melanoma? *J Am Acad Dermatol* 1993; **29**: 989–96.
16. Bataille V, Newton Bishop JA, Sasieni P *et al.* Risk of cutaneous melanoma in relation to the numbers, types and sites of naevi: a case-control study. *Br J Cancer* 1996; **73**: 1605–11.
17. Marghoob AA, Schoenbach SP, Kopf AW *et al.* Large congenital melanocytic nevi and the risk for the development of malignant melanoma. A prospective study. *Arch Dermatol* 1996; **132**: 170–5.
18. Illig L, Weidner F, Hundeiker M *et al.* Congenital nevi ≤ 10 cm as precursors to melanoma: 52 cases, a review, and a new conception. *Arch Dermatol* 1985; **121**: 1274–81.
19. Kefford RF, Newton Bishop JA, Bergman W, Tucker MA. Counseling and DNA testing for individuals perceived to be genetically predisposed to melanoma: a consensus statement of the Melanoma Genetics Consortium. *J Clin Oncol* 1999; **17**: 3245–51.
20. Lederman JS, Sober AJ. Does biopsy type influence survival in clinical stage I cutaneous

melanoma? *J Am Acad Dermatol* 1985; **13**: 983–7.

21. Lees VC, Briggs JC. Effect of initial biopsy procedure on prognosis in Stage 1 invasive cutaneous malignant melanoma: review of 1086 patients. *Br J Surg* 1991; **78**: 1108–10.

22. Austin JR, Byers RM, Brown WD, Wolf P. Influence of biopsy on the prognosis of cutaneous melanoma of the head and neck. *Head Neck* 1996; **18**: 107–17.

23. Association of Directors of Anatomic and Surgical Pathology. Recommendations for the reporting of tissues removed as part of the surgical treatment of cutaneous melanoma. *Pathol Int* 1998; **48**: 168–70.

24. Balch CM, Urist MM, Karakousis CP *et al.* Efficacy of 2-cm surgical margins for intermediate-thickness melanomas (1 to 4 mm): results of a multi-institutional randomized surgical trial. *Ann Surg* 1993; **218**: 262–7.

25. Veronesi U, Cascinelli N, Adamus J *et al.* Thin stage I primary cutaneous malignant melanoma. Comparison of excision with margins of 1 or 3 cm. *N Engl J Med* 1988; **318**: 1159–62.

26. NIH Consensus conference. Diagnosis and treatment of early melanoma. *JAMA* 1992; **268**: 1314–19.

27. Bohler-Sommeregger K, Schuller-Petrovic S, Neumann R, Muller E. Cryosurgery of lentigo maligna. *Plast Reconstr Surg* 1992; **90**: 436–40; discussion 441–4.

28. Mahendran RM, Newton Bishop JA. Survey of U.K. current practice in the treatment of lentigo maligna. *Br J Dermatol* 2001; **144**: 71–6.

29. Schmid-Wendtner MH, Brunner B, Konz B *et al.* Fractionated radiotherapy of lentigo maligna and lentigo maligna melanoma in 64 patients. *J Am Acad Dermatol* 2000; **43**: 477–82.

30. Tsang RW, Liu FF, Wells W, Payne DG. Lentigo maligna of the head and neck. Results of treatment by radiotherapy. *Arch Dermatol* 1994; **130**: 1008–12.

31. McHenry P, MacKie RM. Management of lentigo maligna – cryotherapy versus surgery. *Br J Dermatol* 1994; **131** (Suppl. 44): 15–16.

32. Pitman GH, Kopf AW, Bart RS, Casson PR. Treatment of lentigo maligna and lentigo maligna melanoma. *J Dermatol Surg Oncol* 1979; **5**: 727–37.

33. Coleman WP III, Davis RS, Reed RJ, Krementz ET. Treatment of lentigo maligna and lentigo maligna melanoma. *J Dermatol Surg Oncol* 1980; **6**: 476–9.

34. Lever WF, Schaumburg-Lever G. Melanocytic nevus. In: *Histopathology of the Skin*, 7th edn. Philadelphia: J.B.Lippincott Company, 1990; 756–805.

35. Salopek TG, Slade JM, Marghoob AA *et al.* Management of cutaneous malignant melanoma by dermatologists of the American Academy of Dermatology. II. Definitive surgery for malignant melanoma. *J Am Acad Dermatol* 1995; **33**: 451–61.

36. Timmons MJ. Malignant melanoma excision margins: plastic surgery audit in Britain and Ireland, 1991, and a review. *Br J Plast Surg* 1993; **46**: 525–31.

37. Heaton KM, Sussman JJ, Gershenwald JE *et al.* Surgical margins and prognostic factors in patients with thick (> 4 mm) primary melanoma. *Ann Surg Oncol* 1998; **5**: 322–8.

38. Weedon D. A reappraisal of melanoma *in situ*. *J Dermatol Surg Oncol* 1982; **8**: 774–5.

39. Salman SM, Rogers GS. Prognostic factors in thin cutaneous malignant melanoma. *J Dermatol Surg Oncol* 1990; **16**: 413–18.

40. Basseres N, Grob JJ, Richard MA *et al.* Cost-effectiveness of surveillance of stage I melanoma. A retrospective appraisal based on a 10-year experience in a dermatology department in France. *Dermatology* 1995; **191**: 199–203.

41. Khansur T, Sanders J, Das SK. Evaluation of staging workup in malignant melanoma. *Arch Surg* 1989; **124**: 847–9.

42. Kirkwood JM, Strawderman MH, Ernstoff MS *et al.* Interferon alfa-2b adjuvant therapy of high-risk resected cutaneous melanoma:

the Eastern Cooperative Oncology Group Trial EST 1684. *J Clin Oncol* 1996; **14**: 7–17.

43. Kirkwood JM, Ibrahim JG, Sondak VK *et al.* High- and low-dose interferon alfa-2b in high-risk melanoma: first analysis of intergroup trial E1690/S9111/C9190. *J Clin Oncol* 2000; **18**: 2444–58.

44. Kirkwood JM, Ibrahim JG, Sosman JA *et al.* High-dose interferon alfa-2b significantly prolongs relapse-free and overall survival compared with the GM2-KLH/QS-21 vaccine in patients with resected stage IIB–III melanoma: results of intergroup trial E1694/S9512/C509801. *J Clin Oncol* 2001; **19**: 2370–80.

45. Koops HS, Vaglini M, Suciu S *et al.* Prophylactic isolated limb perfusion for localized, high-risk limb melanoma: results of a multicenter randomized phase III trial. European Organization for Research and Treatment of Cancer Malignant Melanoma Cooperative Group Protocol 18832, the World Health Organization Melanoma Program Trial 15, and the North American Perfusion Group Southwest Oncology Group-8593. *J Clin Oncol* 1998; **16**: 2906–12.

46. Sim FH, Taylor WF, Pritchard DJ, Soule EH. Lymphadenectomy in the management of stage I malignant melanoma: a prospective randomized study. *Mayo Clin Proc* 1986; **61**: 697–705.

47. Cascinelli N, Morabito A, Santinami M *et al.* Immediate or delayed dissection of regional nodes in patients with melanoma of the trunk: a randomised trial. WHO Melanoma Programme. *Lancet* 1998; **351**: 793–6.

48. Morton DL, Wen DR, Wong JH *et al.* Technical details of intraoperative lymphatic mapping for early stage melanoma. *Arch Surg* 1992; **127**: 392–9.

49. Sterne GD, Murray DS, Grimley RP. Ilioinguinal block dissection for malignant melanoma. *Br J Surg* 1995; **82**: 1057–9.

50. Hill S, Thomas JM. Use of the carbon dioxide laser to manage cutaneous metastases from malignant melanoma. *Br J Surg* 1996; **83**: 509–12.

51. Patchell RA, Tibbs PA, Walsh JW *et al.* A randomized trial of surgery in the treatment of single metastases of the brain. *N Engl J Med* 1990; **322**: 494–500.

52. Miller JD. Surgical excision for single cerebral metastasis. *Lancet* 1993; **341**: 1566-7.

53. Peters L, Byers R, Ang K. Radiotherapy for melanoma. In: *Cutaneous Melanoma* (Balch CM, Houghton AN, Milton GW *et al.*, eds), 2nd edn. Philadelphia: Lippincott Williams and Wilkins, 1992; 509–21.

54. Somaza S, Kondziolka D, Lunsford LD *et al.* Stereotactic radiosurgery for cerebral metastatic melanoma. *J Neurosurg* 1993; **79**: 661–6.

55. Ewend MG, Carey LA, Brem H. Treatment of melanoma metastases in the brain. *Semin Surg Oncol* 1996; **12**: 429–35.

56. Falkson CI, Ibrahim J, Kirkwood JM *et al.* Phase III trial of dacarbazine versus dacarbazine with interferon alpha-2b versus dacarbazine with tamoxifen versus dacarbazine with interferon alpha-2b and tamoxifen in patients with metastatic malignant melanoma: an Eastern Cooperative Oncology Group study. *J Clin Oncol* 1998; **16**: 1743–51.

57. Grin CM, Driscoll MS, Grant-Kels JM. Pregnancy and the prognosis of malignant melanoma. *Semin Oncol* 1996; **23**: 734–6.

58. MacKie RM, Bufalino R, Morabito A *et al.* Lack of effect of pregnancy on outcome of melanoma. For The World Health Organisation Melanoma Programme. *Lancet* 1991; **337**: 653–5.

59. Dicker TJ, Kavanagh GM, Herd RM *et al.* A rational approach to melanoma follow-up in patients with primary cutaneous melanoma. Scottish Melanoma Group. *Br J Dermatol* 1999; **140**: 249–54.

60. Balch CM, Buzaid AC, Soong SJ *et al.* Final version of the American Joint Committee on Cancer staging system for cutaneous melanoma. *J Clin Oncol* 2001; **19**: 3635–48.

Table 1
Levels of evidence on which the guideline is based

Level	Type of evidence
Ia	Evidence obtained from meta-analysis of randomized controlled trials
Ib	Evidence obtained from at least one randomized controlled trial
IIa	Evidence obtained from at least one well-designed controlled study without randomization
IIb	Evidence obtained from at least one other type of well-designed quasi-experimental study
III	Evidence obtained from well-designed non-experimental descriptive studies, such as comparative studies, correlation studies and case studies
IV	Evidence obtained from expert committee reports or opinions and/or clinical experience of respected authorities

Grade of recommendation	
A	There is good evidence to support the use of the procedure
B	There is fair evidence to support the use of the procedure
C	There is poor evidence to support the use of the procedure
D	There is fair evidence to support the rejection of the use of the procedure
E	There is good evidence to support the rejection of the use of the procedure

Due to the process of producing unified guidelines, the quality of evidence grading used in these guidelines differs slightly from that used in other British Association of Dermatologists current guidelines; the strength of recommendations grading is the same as used in other publications.

Table 2

The new 2001 American Joint Committee on Cancer (AJCC) staging system

Stage	Primary tumour (pT)	Lymph node (N)	Distant metastases (M)
0	In situ tumours	No nodes	None
IA	< 1.0 mm, no ulceration	No nodes	None
IB	< 1.0 mm with ulceration	No nodes	None
	1.01–2.0 mm, no ulceration	No nodes	None
IIA	1.01–2.0 mm with ulceration	No nodes	None
	2.01–4.0 mm, no ulceration	No nodes	None
IIB	2.01–4.0 mm with ulceration	No nodes	None
	> 4.0 mm, no ulceration	No nodes	None
IIC	> 4.0 mm with ulceration	No nodes	None
IIIA	Any Breslow thickness, no ulceration	Micrometastases in nodes	None
IIIB	Any Breslow thickness with ulceration	Micrometastases in nodes	None
	Any Breslow thickness, no ulceration	Up to three palpable nodes	None
	Any Breslow thickness ± ulceration	No nodes but in-transit metastases or satellites	None
IIIC	Any Breslow thickness with ulceration	Up to three palpable nodes	None
	Any Breslow thickness ± ulceration	Four or more palpable nodes or matted nodes or in-transit metastases with nodes	None
IV			M1: skin, subcutaneous or distant lymph nodes M2: lung M3: all other sites or any site with raised lactate dehydrogenase

The AJCC staging system is recommended for general use.[60]

Appendix 1. Possible audit points for melanoma

- What proportion of lesions had incisional rather than excisional biopsy?
- What proportion of melanomas was seen within 2 weeks of referral?
- If melanomas have been excised in general practice but not referred...
- Audit completeness of clinical and/or pathology data recording compared with the guidelines dataset

- Audit treatment modalities used for lentigo maligna melanoma
- Have patients had appropriate investigations according to stage of melanoma, and what are the results for each investigation?
- Have eligible patients been counselled about clinical trials, and what proportion has been entered?
- For patients entering clinical trials, have entry criteria been fulfilled (e.g. adequate number of lymph nodes examined pathologically after a block dissection)?

Index

Note: 'vs' indicated differentiation of two conditions. Abbreviations: BCC, basal cell carcinoma; MM, malignant melanoma; SCC, squamous cell carcinoma.